Natural Healing with
*A*romatherapy

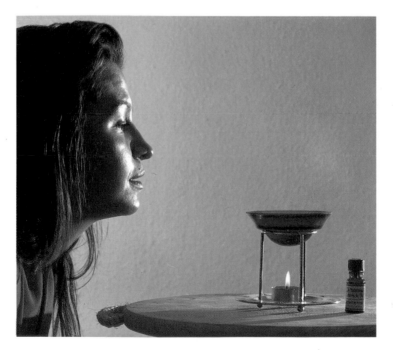

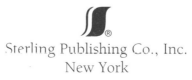

Sterling Publishing Co., Inc.
New York

Library of Congress Cataloging-in-Publication Data Available

10 9 8 7 6 5 4 3 2 1

Published by Sterling Publishing
Company, Inc.
387 Park Avenue South, New York,
N.Y. 10016
Originally Published in Germany under
the title *Natürliche Heilung durch
Aromatherapie,* 4th printing 1977 and
© 1995 by Gräfe und Unzer Verlag
GmbH, München
English Translation © 1999 by Sterling
Publishing Co., Inc.
Distributed in Canada by Sterling
Publishing
C/o Canadian Manda Group,
One Atlantic Avenue, Suite 105
Toronto, Ontario
Canada M6K 3E7
Distributed in Great Britain and Europe
by Cassell PLC
Wellington House, 125 Strand
London WC2R 0BB, England
Distributed in Australia by Capricorn
Link (Australia) Pty Ltd.
P.O. Box 6651, Baulkham Hills
Business Centre, NSW 2153,
Australia

Printed in Hong Kong
All rights reserved

Sterling ISBN 0-8069-4221-5

Contents

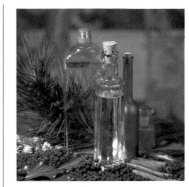

The healing powers of chamomile are almost legendary. The essential oil of this plant should be in everyone's medicine cabinet.

Preface

Scents can give you inspiration, improve your health, and grant you an inner sense of harmony. Some stimulate and refresh, whereas others have a calming and relaxing effect. You can really perform magic with scents; you can calm down if you are angry, forget your sorrows, and chase away fear and pain. Just put a few drops of rose oil or neroli oil into your essence burner, and anger and nervousness will vanish. Headaches can be combated with peppermint or sage oil. Essential oils can also be used for stomach ailments, troubled sleep, lumbago, and skin problems.

Good, pure scents are not only pleasant, but they can also have a deep effect on the mind and the body.

External and Internal Usage

Essential oils are absorbed through the olfactory sense, which reacts faster than any of the other senses. They are also absorbed through the skin when used in baths and massages, as well as in creams, compresses, facial toner, and perfumes. The subject of ingesting essential oils is controversial, because the effects on the sensitive stomach lining have not been researched sufficiently. Therefore, I generally don't recommend using aroma oils orally. To find out what you need to look out for when using specific oils and mixing particular essences, refer to the chapter "Tips for the Correct Use of Aroma Oils."

Inhaling Scents for Immediate Effects

Scents work most effectively when they are inhaled. They arrive directly in the cerebrum by way of the limbic system. This is why the effect is almost instantaneous. For example, you smell a rose, a smile crosses your face, and you feel instantly so much better. Inhaling peppermint oil when you have a headache can produce a similar effect.

If used in baths, essential oils travel through the pores of the skin to the muscles, the joints, all internal organs, and, most importantly, the endocrine glands, where they encourage and accelerate the healing process.

You Still Have to See Your Doctor . . .

Where serious illnesses are concerned, using essential oils, of course, cannot replace a visit to the doctor. In these cases, aromatherapy should be understood as a supplementary measure, to alleviate acute complaints, to improve general well-being, and, most importantly, to strengthen the body's power to fight off disease. Especially Australian tea tree oil, but also oils like rosemary and thyme, kill bacteria, viruses, and fungi, as well as reduce the risk of infection.

Same Oil—Different Effects

Don't be surprised if the same essential oil is recommended for a number of different uses over the course of this book. Many of the oils have a very broad spectrum, and can be beneficial in more than one respect. This is because the oils are composed of a multitude of different active ingredients. Rosemary oil, for example, improves memory and concentration, fights infectious diseases, encourages hair growth, improves eyesight, stimulates the appetite, and lowers cholesterol levels.

Using aromatherapy oils shouldn't tempt you to omit necessary visits to your doctor. And many doctors today have an open-minded attitude toward alternative medicine.

Essential oils always work in a comprehensive manner, and their effects show themselves in different areas. Aroma oils are therefore extremely versatile.

Essential Oils—an Overview

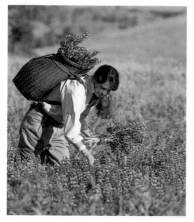

A walk through a summer meadow filled with flowers is very pleasant. Essential oils made from flowers allow you to enjoy your favorite scents at home too.

Essential oils are obtained through steam distillation, whereas essences are the product of a pressurizing process. Also, there is a process whereby solvents are used to obtain scents from plants.

Scents play a much greater role in our lives than you may have realized. They help us remember and recognize events from our past, and affect the way that we, often instinctively, judge a situation. The smell of a wooden pencil may remind you of your schooldays (evoking either positive or negative memories). Your mother's or father's scent, or the fresh smell of a forest, may bring back memories of family outings.

It has also been discovered that we are led by scents—a fact that is exploited by the advertising industry. Scents are used, for example, in department stores at a level that the human brain doesn't notice consciously. Increases in sales, however, have proven that the advertisers had the right idea.

Perfumes, too, bring forth associations. For instance, the heavier, sensual musk scents are associated with sexuality, the lighter, fresh and fruity scents with innocence, and the herbal, earthy scents with nature and naturalness.

Manufacture and Quality

Essential oils are obtained through a process of distillation and subsequent cooling, which separates the oil, which floats on top, from the water. The water doesn't go to waste, but is used, for example, in facial toners and bubble baths.

Some plants have to be treated with solvents to filter out the aromatic substance, which is then separated from the solvent in the second stage of the process. There is, however, always a small risk of traces of the solvent remaining behind in the oil. Therefore, these oils must never be used internally!

Only use genuine, pure essential oils, because just these will have the desired effects. There are now a lot of synthetic oils and oil blends on the market, which are often sold as "natural essential oils." They are usually less expensive, but not as effective. Always be sure to buy pure essential oils, and consult the salesperson or the manufacturer of the oil if this isn't specified on the package.

A few drops of the essential oil are usually enough. Essential oils should only be applied to the skin diluted—that is, 1 to 2 percent of the essential oil blended with a carrier oil.

How to Use Essential Oils

Essential oils are highly concentrated, so they are almost always used diluted in either water or a carrier oil. Be sure to read the instructions for dosage.

If you wish to scent a room, use between 5 and 15 drops in the essence burner. Use the same amount in a hot bath, once the water has filled the tub. For a body or massage oil, add 10 to 20 drops of the concentrate to the body oil. All cold-pressed oils, such as jojoba, almond, and avocado oil, are suitable as body oils. For compresses, you will only need to use 2 to 3 drops of oil, mixed in no more than a pint (half a liter) of warm water. For seasoning food, blend no more than 3 drops of the oil with cold-pressed thistle oil, which has a fairly neutral flavor and brings out the aroma of the oil. In the sauna, 5 drops of oil per ladle of water are sufficient.

The water that remains after distillation is rich in aromatic substances. However, many of the perfumes available in stores are simply a blend of water with essential or synthetic oils.

Harmonizing Scents

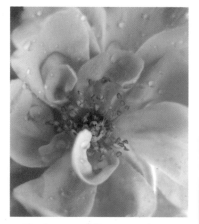

The "queen of flowers" releases a harmonizing scent, which will also lift moods and give joy when captured in an essential oil.

Aroma oils have a powerful effect not only on the body but also on the mind. They can help you achieve, maintain, and strengthen your emotional balance. With regular use, you will notice how energized and well you will feel. And with this positive emotional foundation, you will be much less susceptible to illness.

For Inner Balance

In order to regain inner balance, it's important to try to eliminate negative circumstances and character traits. For this, however, you will need a clear mind and a willingness to confront certain problems. In this section, you will find lists of oils that counteract negative influences, and thus help you achieve an inner calm.

Fear

Fear of exams, excitement over a trip, and shock are best treated with 2 to 3 drops of lavender, neroli, peppermint, angelica, or basil on a handkerchief.

The following oils are useful in combating fear: benzoin, geranium, chamomile, patchouli, sandalwood, and ylang-ylang. Use them in baths, in massage oils, in your essence burner, and when you create your own perfumes (see the chapter "Tips for the Correct Use of Aroma Oils"). Inhaling directly from the scent bottle is the best method for alleviating an acute attack of fear.

Scent your bedroom with lavender, neroli, petitgrain, or sandalwood to avoid having troubling nightmares. Of course, you can always mix these oils. Angst can be driven away with angelica, honey, rose, and pine, especially if the angst is without foundation. Follow your nose in aromatherapy, deciding for yourself which of these oils you prefer. If you don't find a particular scent pleasant, then it probably won't have the desired effect on you.

Anger

At the end of a long and exhausting day, it may take very little to make you angry, and that's it, there's no hope of having a badly needed relaxing evening. Try to counteract this negative state by creating a calming, mood-lifting atmosphere with the help of geranium, melissa, neroli, rose, or cedar. If you would like to create a gently eroticizing ambience to detract further from your anger, also add a few drops of patchouli or ylang-ylang (or the less costly cananga).

Depression

People who suffer from depression often don't have the emotional strength to do what is best for them, and friends and family will have to lend a helping hand. Fortunately, there are a number of essential oils that will help someone with emotional difficulties regain hope and self-confidence. However, these should not be used just occasionally, but consistently over a period of time. It's particularly important that those suffering from depression choose the aroma oils they prefer themselves, because they will know instinctively what they need and what is good for them. There is a wide choice, from bergamot, geranium, jasmine, and lavender to melissa, rose, yarrow, and tonka bean to violet, ylang-ylang, lemon, and stone pine.

TIP
If you are in a state of fear, add equal amounts of melissa and basil to your essence burner.

Scents influence both the body and the soul, and can help you gain inner calm, heal illnesses, and improve your overall sense of well-being.

When treating depression and other emotional problems, it's important to find a scent that fosters your sense of well-being. There is such a wide choice of aroma oils that you should be able to discover a scent that is especially to your liking.

How to Rid Yourself of Negative Thoughts

🌣 Always carry a scent bottle, preferably filled with neroli.

🌣 Only use skin-care products that effuse your chosen healing scent.

🌣 Before you go to bed, take a bath using a mood-lifting aroma oil.

🌣 Use your chosen aroma to scent your wardrobe and your linen cupboard.

Overcoming Depression with Neroli

No other oil, however, can treat depression as effectively as neroli can. Neroli is the oil obtained from the blossoms of the bitter orange tree. Unfortunately, it is very costly, and can only be purchased in the smallest amounts: To distill 1 kilogram of the essential oil, approximately 1,000 kilograms of the blossom are needed. The flowery scent has a strong calming effect, and chases away negative thoughts. It is too precious to be used in the essence burner, but diluting it with jojoba oil works very well, and the beautiful characteristic scent is retained.

TIP
To dilute neroli, add the jojoba oil directly to the neroli bottle. Shake well and check repeatedly to see if the scent of neroli still pervades strongly enough.

If depressions are so severe that a person feels completely trapped, the use of essential oils cannot replace the skills of a qualified counselor or psychotherapist. However, aromatherapy can improve one's general frame of mind, and may even help prevent an emotional crisis, if only in the short term. Therefore, don't despair if you are feeling low, because you might receive an unexpected lift from essential oils.

Neroli also combines well with bergamot oil, which gives Earl Grey tea its characteristic aroma, and itself has a refreshing, mood-lifting effect.

Indecision

Should I or shouldn't I? People about to make an important decision will ask themselves that question. But if you are one of those people who ponder even the smallest matter long and hard, and in the end still can't make up your mind, then you will find eucalyptus, clary sage, rosemary, and lemon of particular benefit. These essential oils boost our confidence and give us the courage to try something new.

Exhaustion

To overcome nervous exhaustion, aromatherapy uses angelica, cajeput, camphor, peppermint, rosemary, and lemon. Again, inhaling the aroma directly from your scent bottle may be the best method.

Physical exhaustion, on the other hand, is best treated with basil, rosemary, ginger, marjoram, clove, thyme, and juniper. I personally have experienced the best results with basil and rosemary. However, any of these scents, added to the bath or the essence burner, or used in massages or straight from the bottle, work like a fountain of youth, and are refreshing and revitalizing.

But you must not rely on the beneficial effects of these oils alone. If you are chronically exhausted, you need to "switch off" from your worries at home or at work, and find time to relax, otherwise a breakdown might be inevitable. Enjoying a short break in a beautiful spot, like a green park flooded with sunlight, combined with aromatherapy treatment, will soon restore your mental and physical balance.

The eucalyptus tree needs large amounts of water. Therefore, it was planted in Europe to dry out swamps, thus robbing the mosquito of its habitat. Eucalyptus also activates the red blood cells and increases the supply of oxygen to the body. So, if you are suffering from apathy and listlessness, the fresh scent of eucalyptus will have a reviving and motivating effect on you. In addition, its antiseptic properties render it useful in treating colds and wounds.

TIP
If you are feeling physically exhausted, add equal parts of marjoram, clove, and sage to your essence burner.

Lack of Concentration

Rosemary is especially helpful if you have trouble concentrating. Basil, bay, myrtle, peppermint, and lemon produce a similar effect. Peppermint, in particular, refreshes the mind and strengthens mental powers. Just add a few drops to your essence burner or to your handkerchief, and you will find it much easier to stay focused.

Sorrow

Benzoin, bergamot, jasmine, marjoram, peru balsam, rose, and sandalwood will comfort you, and are very well suited to help you deal with sorrow, whatever its cause. Benzoin, jasmine, and rose are especially suited to children who have suffered a great loss, whereas adults who have lost someone close may react better to marjoram and bergamot. Rosemary is also helpful in giving solace to the bereaved, and in giving them a new faith in the future.

Listlessness

Know the feeling? You have the time and would like to get a few things accomplished, but can't make up your mind what to do. You just potter around without much enthusiasm, and later on feel annoyed at yet another wasted opportunity. Ginger, lemongrass, thyme, and lemon give us the strength to overcome this listlessness.

Feelings of Inferiority

Feelings of inferiority can be experienced to varying degrees. Some people only notice them occasionally—for example, on congratulating a close friend on an achievement and having to admit to themselves, some-

Peppermint oil is cooling and refreshing, and improves memory and concentration. Whether used at home or at work, peppermint will help to clear your mind, allowing your thoughts to flow again.

If listlessness takes over, it's advisable to bathe, massage, or change the room ambience with one of the appropriate scents.

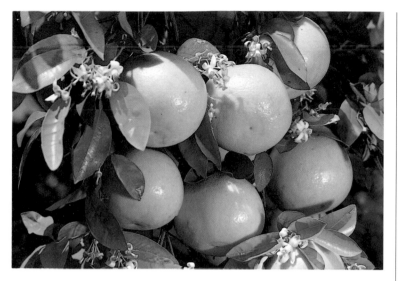

what enviously, that they could never perform the same feat. In cases like this, a few drops of geranium, jasmine, rose, or ylang-ylang will suffice, and the balance is restored.

Other people, however, suffer from a life-long inferiority complex, and every little misfortune they undergo serves as proof that they have indeed failed in life and will forevermore. Often the root causes for such misconceptions and lack of self-esteem are buried in a person's early childhood, so it's best to consult a good therapist to try to come to terms with the formative experiences upon which they are based.

Tiredness

Tiredness may be a signal sent by your body, indicating that it simply needs a break. If possible, you should allow yourself one; but, if not, then you may wish to use basil, marjoram, clove, rosemary, or thyme to revive your spirits.

If you are exhausted or merely tired, a refreshing bath will revive you. Add some rosemary oil to the bath water, and just relax. The spicy, fresh scent has a stimulating effect on the nervous system, and improves circulation.

However, don't try to outsmart your body and push it continuously to its limits. This could have dire consequences, possibly leading to a serious illness.

Nervousness

Often nervousness is related to actual stress, but it can also be caused by a relative weakness of the nervous system. This is why sometimes people are nervous and jittery even if there is no reason for them to feel stressed. Such cases call for long-term treatment with valerian, bergamot, chamomile, lavender, marjoram, or sandalwood. These oils can be combined in whichever way you prefer, but they also release their beneficial powers when used individually. You can add them to your essence burner or use them in baths or skin-care products.

Valerian, bergamot, chamomile, lavender, marjoram, and sandalwood strengthen the nervous system, and can calm people who are irritable. Their fresh, strong scents create a sense of inner harmony and a relaxed atmosphere.

Despondency

If you tend to feel that the world is a cheerless place, and can't see the faintest glimmer of hope on the horizon, jasmine, lavender, and ylang-ylang will brighten your life.

TIP
If you can't seem to rid yourself of feelings of despondency, treat yourself to a bath, adding 8 drops of lavender, 3 drops of jasmine, and 4 drops of ylang-ylang.

Emotional Dependence

Essential oils aid the process of liberating the self. To overcome emotional dependence, feelings of inadequacy, and negative moods, use juniper for support. Bergamot, jasmine, rose, and sandalwood raise courage and self-confidence. Massages achieve the best results for deeply rooted feelings of inferiority, but baths are helpful, too, as is the scenting of rooms and personal care products.

There are two more oils that work in a similar way: bay and thuja. *However, they are highly toxic and must never be used internally.* Thuja can cause kidney damage, and is entirely unsuitable for children. Care should be taken even when using these oils externally in massages or baths. They should only be used following the advice of an experienced therapist.

Stress

In this day and age, almost everyone is plagued by some degree of stress. Youngsters in kindergarten have to deal with it, and pensioners may have retired from their jobs, but still aren't entirely free of stress. Noise is everywhere, a great hustle and bustle. Unfortunately, not being able to cope with stress will weaken our resistance to all manner of disease.

To overcome everyday stress, regular baths using angelica, honey, chamomile, lavender, melissa, neroli, rose, or rosemary are beneficial. In stressful situations, it also helps to open your scent bottle and smell the aroma directly.

More Ways to Combat Stress

❀ Eat a light diet, rich in vitamins, with plenty of fruit, salads, and fresh vegetables.

❀ Take regular breaks while you are at work.

❀ Eat regular meals, and take your time over them.

❀ Get plenty of sleep.

Baths and massages will improve the way you feel about your body. Bergamot, jasmine, rose, and sandalwood help reduce feelings of inferiority and emotional dependence. If you treat yourself to a bath or a massage with one of these essential oils, you will be able to face the day refreshed and revitalized.

Your first step in fighting stress is to have the determination not to be governed by it. Angelica, honey, chamomile, lavender, melissa, neroli, rose, and rosemary all help combat stress; use them in the bath or, for an acute attack, straight from the scent bottle.

TIP
If you are undecided and feeling lethargic, add equal parts of lime, grapefruit, and rosemary to your essence burner.

Lethargy

People suffering from lethargy give the impression of being constantly sleepy, uninterested, and apathetic. Strong revitalizing oils are necessary to "awaken" these people, but it's important not to use too much.

Pepper oil can work magic in these cases, but it can unfortunately often lead to skin irritations. However, if used in an essence burner, it will cause no side effects. Other oils that are recommended are citronella, lime, thyme, cinnamon, and lemon.

Benzoin and the warm, sweet smell of honey are like a tonic for over-wrought nerves. But if you prefer a drier aroma, use styrax instead.

Irritability

Constant irritability should not be taken lightly. If everything annoys and irritates you, this needs to be addressed right away. What others may consider to be just a grouchy mood can, in the people concerned, lead to both physical and emotional illnesses. Benzoin, honey, and styrax provide quick help in lessening irritability.

Lack of Assertiveness

Less assertive people tend to allow others to lead the way. They don't always do this happily, however, because they know that they often act against their better judgment and do things that they know aren't right or good for them. Nevertheless, they seem to be incapable of opposing an argument or a seemingly convincing decision made by someone else.

If you often feel like a puppet, angelica, oregano, rosemary, sage, and cypress will strengthen your resolve and self-confidence, giving you a greater ability to succeed in

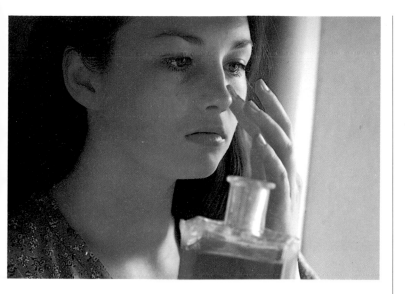

Rosemary and thyme are the most popular choices for overcoming physical exhaustion. They can be used in your essence burner, added to your bath, or dissolved in your facial toner—the decision is yours.

REMEDY:

A REGENERATING
MASSAGE OIL:

Blend 15 drops of ginger and 5 drops each of rosemary and lemongrass with 50 ml of almond oil. Shake well. Use to massage the upper body, back, and legs.

your intentions. Try them out, and don't give up immediately if you don't see instant results. Eventually, you are sure to be successful.

For Your General Well-being

You can greatly improve your overall sense of well-being if you scent your rooms with your favorite aromas. These will constantly, though almost imperceptibly, stimulate your olfactory nerves, which transport the aroma to your body. In this section, you will find harmonizing scents for your general well-being. Would you like your home to smell like a flower garden, a spring meadow, or a fresh sea breeze? Should it carry the scent of exotic spices, a dark forest, or succulent fruit? Would you like a scent reminiscent of a tale from the *Arabian Nights?* This is entirely up to you. What follow are a few blends that you can add to the water in your essence burner.

Essential oils can be used in your essence burner to improve your sense of emotional well-being, and to heal respiratory tract complaints, such as colds, coughs, and hoarseness.

"Flower Garden"

- ✤ 2 drops of rose
- ✤ 1 drop of jasmine
- ✤ 2 drops of lavender
- ✤ 2 drops of ylang-ylang

"Spring Meadow"

- ✤ 2 drops of bergamot
- ✤ 2 drops of lemongrass
- ✤ 3 drops of palmarosa
- ✤ 2 drops of pine
- ✤ 2 drops of violet
- ✤ A little citronella spray

"Arabian Nights"

- ✤ 2 drops of elemi
- ✤ 2 drops of cananga
- ✤ 2 drops of ambrette seed
- ✤ 2 drops of myrrh
- ✤ 2 drops of patchouli
- ✤ 2 drops of sandalwood

It is usually sufficient to use three of the oils in the blends above. However, you can experiment using all six, and, in addition, spray your room with ylang-ylang.

"Sea Breeze"

- ✤ 2 drops of peppermint
- ✤ 2 drops of petitgrain
- ✤ 2 drops of lime
- ✤ 2 drops of palmarosa

The scent of a mix of exotic spices conveys a feeling of warmth and security. You can choose from anise, benzoin, ginger, cardamom, clary sage, nutmeg, clove, and cinnamon. Use them in any combination in your essence burner—they all go together well.

Fresh "Forest Air," created with the essential oils of silver fir, fir, pine, stone pine, and cypress, is bliss if you have a cold or trouble with your bronchial tubes or lungs. Add an interesting hint of orange oil, which you can also use in room sprays. Pine needle oil helps in soothing insect bites and sunburn.

Ambrette seed is the natural substitute for the synthetic musk scent used in the perfume industry. Ambrette seed oil is obtained from the seeds of the hibiscus plant, and has a pleasantly warm and slightly sweet scent.

A "Fruity Melange" is especially popular with children, and can be enhanced and finished by adding a little honey and vanilla oil.

There is nothing like the essential oils of grapefruit, lime, mandarin, orange, and lemon to lift negative moods.

Combining Scents and Colors

Remember that colors can also influence your frame of mind. The "Sea Breeze" formula works best with cool blues and greens. The "Flower Garden" blend will thrive with shades of pink and lilac, and exotic spices develop their full bouquet with gentle shades of ochre and brown. The "Spring Meadow" mixture inspires images of light yellows and greens, and the seducing scents of "Arabian Nights" are best enjoyed with dark reds and purples.

Although scents and colors obviously affect different senses, they have a lot in common. They can be mixed and blended in innumerable ways, creating different nuances and evoking various emotions.

Aromatherapy can be used in conjunction with other therapies, such as aura-soma therapy, which uses colors. In all cultures and religions, specific colors are associated with feelings of physical and emotional well-being.

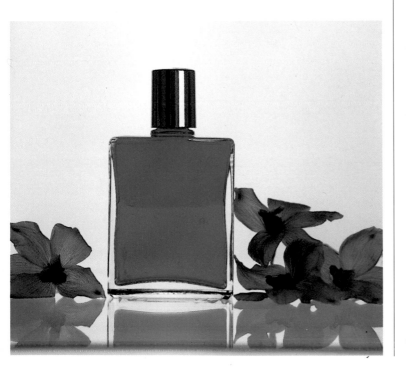

By creating your personal perfume, you can wear your own individual scent.

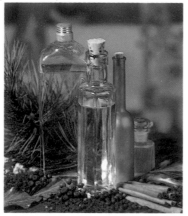

Spices have long been known for their healing properties

Healing Physical Complaints

Among the properties of many essential oils is the capacity to fight bacteria and viruses. In addition, some oils can lessen pain, reduce temperature, strengthen the body's immune system, or reduce the risk of infection.

The ancient art of healing made use of these amazing properties. Healing herbs were gathered and dried, and then the essential oils were distilled by means of a very complex method, to be used in ointments, tinctures, and pills. This ancient knowledge is experiencing a revival today in alternative medicine.

Allergies

Allergies have become some of the most frequently voiced complaints in modern society. An allergy is the excessive reaction to certain substances, situations, or physical states that are without comparable effect on the average person. Of course, allergies have to be investigated by a doctor to determine their cause. There are, however, certain oils that have proven to be beneficial in treating them.

If you are suffering from an allergy to dust mites, you can use tea tree oil as a natural disinfectant in your home. When you mop the floor, add about 50 drops of tea tree oil to the water, or add a few drops to your humidifier or essence burner. Rose oil provides relief from hay fever, whereas tea tree oil and lavender alleviate itching if you suffer from neurodermatitis.

If you suffer from hay fever, but cannot tolerate rose oil, try using chamomile, eucalyptus, lavender, or melissa instead.

Chronic Illnesses

Alleviating pain and improving a person's overall sense of well-being are especially important where chronic illnesses are concerned. Oils, such as bergamot, geranium, jasmine, lavender, lemongrass, neroli, and ylang-ylang, can be recommended as mood-lifters. Having the correct room climate (temperature and humidity) and inhaling from the scent bottle can instill hope and courage, which in turn will increase the patient's ability to cope with the special circumstances of his or her illness. The willingness alone to try something new is a good sign. Only if you give up on yourself will you be taken over by the pain and the suffering.

Asthma

If you suffer from asthma, you shouldn't inhale essential oils from the essence burner, because humid warmth is not good for asthmatics. It is preferable to spray essential oils or to use them in the diffuser or on the aroma stone. In cases of an acute attack, inhaling the scent straight from the scent bottle helps initially; then the treatment is continued with rubs administered to the entire upper body.

The same healing oils recommended for asthma (see sidebar) also fight a stubborn cough. In this case, inhaling from the bottle is the most effective option, and gentle rubs of the neck and the chest with the respective massage oil are beneficial as well (see "Tips for the Correct Use of Aroma Oils").

Blood Pressure—Too High or Too Low

If your blood pressure is too low, massages and baths with camphor, peppermint, rosemary, sage, thyme, and hyssop

The most effective oils for asthma are anise, benzoin, bergamot, chamomile, lavender, neroli, thyme, frankincense, and hyssop.

The strong, honey-like scent of rosemary has a warming and stimulating effect on the heart and blood circulation. You can use it in your essence burner, in the bath, or to make tea. Its stimulating, antispasmodic, and nerve-strengthening properties made it popular in ancient Greece and Rome.

Lemon oil, used externally, causes potassium carbonate to be produced in the body. This will then neutralize an excess of acids, and will even help wash out uric acid, which accumulates in the joints, and can thus prevent gout.

IMPORTANT
Do not use hyssop if you are epileptic or if you are pregnant.

Lavender has anti-spasmodic, anti-inflammatory, and regenerating properties, and it improves circulation. Dissolve 12 to 15 drops of lavender oil in a little milk, and add this to the bath water.

will help to raise it. High blood pressure can be lowered with basil, garlic (also fresh), lavender, marjoram, melissa, neroli, and ylang-ylang. Rosemary, by the way, has the amazing ability of normalizing blood pressure, and can be used for both high and low blood pressure. However, with high blood pressure, use it only occasionally and sparingly.

Gout

Gout is a metabolic disease, marked by a painful inflammation of the joints. Gout can be healed, but unfortunately it can also turn into a chronic illness. The inflammation of the joints is caused by uric acid, which gathers in the joints in the form of crystals. If you have gout, you need to detoxify your body, and warm baths and rubs with angelica, fennel, juniper, lemon, and/or cypress will stimulate this detoxification. To improve circulation, which facilitates the removal of toxins, use hot compresses with ginger, marjoram, or black pepper oil. The pain can be reduced with baths, cold and warm compresses, and rubs with benzoin, chamomile, lavender, rosemary, and tea tree. Move the joints as much as possible after a heat treatment with essential oils, to keep the heat from accumulating in them.

Rheumatism

If you suffer from rheumatism, you probably know how soothing heat is. Baths with chamomile, lavender, marjoram, nutmeg, rosemary, juniper, and/or cypress reduce pain and improve circulation, as well as help to detoxify the body. If you are in acute pain, then hot compresses with lavender or rosemary are recommended too. However, these hot compresses can be harmful in the long run, because they can easily cause heat to accumulate in the joints. For rheumatism, massages with essential oils are indispensable due to their capacity to increase blood circulation. Rubs can be helpful as well.

With all chronic illnesses, it is essential to make changes in your lifestyle in areas that may have brought forth the disease—for example,

∞ reduce (or eliminate) your intake of alcohol, nicotine, and caffeine,

∞ eat more fresh foods,

∞ eat less meat (preferably none),

∞ drink herbal teas, and

∞ exercise in the open air as much as possible.

A daily walk lasting 45 minutes can ease complaints considerably.

Eating Disorders and Weight Problems

Both women and men are affected by eating disorders and weight problems. Not only does vanity play a role, but health concerns are an issue as well. Someone who is overweight is more prone to many diseases, but an exaggerated desire to be slim and a constant lack of appetite will surely lead to health problems after a certain time too.

Lack of Appetite and Bouts of Excessive Eating

A lack of appetite can have numerous causes. Often it occurs after a long illness, during convalescence. It can be brought on by grief and worries, but also by being in love. People react differently to emotional strains: Fear and stress cause eating bouts in some, but lead others to refuse food altogether.

IMPORTANT
In the case of infectious diseases, always consult your doctor.

In treating a lack of appetite, the most effective essential oils are tarragon, ginger, cardamom, caraway, nutmeg, and oregano. They are suitable for use in baths, massage oils, and scent bottles, as well as in creating a better room climate. They will also stimulate the appetite if used, in combination with lemon, as seasoning in cooking.

IMPORTANT
Fennel oil must never be used on children under six years of age. Give them fennel honey or fennel tea instead.

Fennel oil can have a balancing effect, because it can curb the appetite as well as stimulate it. Roman soldiers used to chew fennel seeds on their endless marches so that they wouldn't feel hungry. Similarly, bergamot oil is used primarily to stimulate the appetite, but it can also curb a pathological desire to eat. Both fennel and bergamot are used for baths, massages, scenting personal body-care products, and creating the appropriate room climate.

Anorexia

In young girls who strive to fit the ultra-thin ideal in our society, or perhaps subconsciously fight the natural process of becoming a woman, anorexia can turn into a life-threatening disorder. For them, treatment by a good psychotherapist is therefore essential. As an adjunct to psychotherapy, aromatherapy offers treatment with essential oils in the form of baths and massages. Once the patient has discovered her favorite oils, she should also scent her room with them, as well as her perfume and her skin-care products. Rose is always a good choice. (See "Tips for the Correct Use of Aroma Oils.")

The most effective essential oils for treating anorexia are bergamot, chamomile, neroli, geranium, lavender, rose, jasmine, clary sage, and ylang-ylang. They improve the patient's overall sense of well-being and help her accept her body again.

The previously mentioned oils do not merely stimulate the appetite, but, more importantly, they work on the psyche. They help the patient see her own body in a more positive light, boost her self-confidence, and assist her in overcoming fears and stress, and they also have a calming and warming effect, in addition to antidepressant properties. Particularly at the beginning of their treatment, anorexics will need a lot of vitamins and minerals, especially zinc. Fruit, raw vegetables, and salads are the most likely foods to be accepted by anorexics, because they aren't fattening, and they will at least supply the most important nutrients to the body.

Obesity and Its Treatment

1

Because their olfactory sense is often not working properly, obese people first of all need to be given massages with a carrier oil to which bergamot, fennel, geranium, rosemary, juniper, lemon, and/or cypress have been added (see "Tips for the Correct Use of Aroma Oils").

2

This blend of aroma oils should also be used in baths.

3

Eating a lot of garlic and onions will support the function of the thyroid gland, which is important for regulating body weight.

4

Fennel helps to curb the appetite. It is preferable to chew the seeds and drink a lot of strong fennel tea.

5

Juniper has a strong diuretic effect, and therefore frees the body from waste products. However, high dosages of juniper are not recommended—a few drops are sufficient. High dosages may easily produce the opposite effect to the one desired.

Fennel strengthens the stomach and helps to dampen hunger. Whether inhaled as a scent or used as a tea or an oil, fennel therefore curbs the appetite and the desire to eat.

Obesity

Obesity is possibly more difficult to cure with aromatherapy, because the olfactory sense in overweight people tends to be not as well developed as in others. However, some aromatherapists have had very good results with bergamot, which is an excellent mood-lifter, regulates the appetite, and chases away depression.

Skin Complaints

Dermatologists are of the opinion that about a third of all skin disorders and irritations have a psychosomatic cause.

Basil, lemongrass, melissa, peppermint, thyme, and lemon oils can irritate the skin.

The Most Effective Essential Oils for Skin Problems

ACNE

Facial toner: Use bergamot, geranium, and lavender. Facial oil: Use evening primrose oil as a carrier, and add geranium, rosemary, and sandalwood. Face pack (2 to 3 times a week): Add some water to 3 tablespoons of healing earth to make it into a thin paste; then stir in 1 drop of bergamot, 2 drops of geranium, 1 drop of chamomile, and 1 drop of cypress.

Subsequent treatment: wheat germ oil with lavender and neroli.

ECZEMA

Baths and massages or rubs with chamomile, lavender, tea tree, hyssop, and cedar. To a moisturizing-cream base, add lavender, tea tree, juniper, and frankincense, and for dry eczema, add geranium.

HERPES

For blisters around the lips, alternately apply undiluted lavender and a blend of melissa and tea tree oil on 1 teaspoon of alcohol.

For herpes in the genital area, pour the same blend into 1 quart, or liter, of boiled water and shake vigorously. Use this to wash the affected areas frequently.

DERMATITIS (noninfectious)

Facial toner: Use geranium, chamomile, neroli, and sandalwood. Facial or body oil: Use aloe vera, jojoba, or evening primrose as carrier oils; then add benzoin, immortelle, chamomile, lavender, neroli, and sandalwood.

Take lukewarm baths with chamomile, lavender, and myrtle.

FURUNCLE

Apply hot compresses with bergamot, chamomile, and lavender. Wash the surrounding area with the above oils and heavily diluted onion oil.

ITCHING

Don't scratch! This can cause inflammations and eczema. Apply 1 to 2 drops of undiluted lavender or tea tree oil. Baths with 3 drops of lavender and 3 drops of chamomile are also very helpful, especially just before bedtime. Cold washes are useful in between. Blend one or two of the above oils with 1 teaspoon of alcohol, and pour into half a quart, or liter, of boiled water.

Alternative oils are melissa, peppermint, and sandalwood.

ULCERS

Apply warm compresses with benzoin, bergamot, lavender, niaouli, and tea tree.

Wash the surrounding area frequently with these oils (cold washes).

SHINGLES

With a brush or a cotton swab, apply undiluted bergamot, eucalyptus, or tea tree several times daily. In the evening, take an aroma bath with the same oils.

Subsequent treatment: chamomile and lavender.

The Most Effective Essential Oils for Skin Problems

SCAB (on the head)

Apply about 1 ounce, or 30 grams, of cream base, blended with 12 drops of lavender, 6 drops of myrrh, and 12 drops of tea tree oil, four times daily.

Subsequent treatment with rosemary water will encourage new hair growth.

FUNGAL DISEASES

If the skin is moist and oozing, apply citronella, chamomile, lavender, myrrh, peppermint, and tea tree, dissolved in pure alcohol. Once the skin has become drier, blend your chosen oils with an ointment base and continue the treatment.

For athlete's foot, also use thyme and tea tree footbaths

WARTS

They aren't just disfiguring, but can also be quite painful, especially when they appear on the soles of the feet. The best remedy is undiluted lemon oil, applied with a cotton swab.

For subsequent treatment, blend wheat germ oil with some lavender and rub on. Garlic, taken as capsules or fresh, will accelerate the healing process.

SCABIES

Baths with chamomile, lavender, and rosemary, twice daily. After the bath, apply an ointment base with 5 percent bergamot, lavender, melissa, peppermint, and/or lemon, as well as 2 to 3 drops of either clove or cinnamon.

Subsequent treatment for dried-out skin: Blend any carrier oil with benzoin, lavender, myrrh, or neroli. It's advisable to take garlic at the same time, either in capsules or fresh.

PSORIASIS

Very difficult to cure. British aromatherapist Tisserand has had success with the following remedy. First apply compresses with chamomile and lavender only, then add bergamot, and in the third phase also add geranium. In addition, take baths with these four oils. Regular rubs with evening primrose oil as the carrier oil, blended with bergamot, cajeput, labdanum, immortelle, oregano, and/or tea tree, will alleviate symptoms.

In some cases, good results have been achieved by alternately applying undiluted tea tree oil and tea tree oil combined with the above carrier oil or a corresponding cream.

CELLULITE

Baths and massages with fennel, chamomile, orange, oregano, grapefruit, rosemary, yarrow, juniper, lemon, and/or cypress. For baths, blend 3 drops each of four of the above oils with 2 tablespoons of runny honey. The same blend is also suitable as a massage oil. Juniper is very important in this treatment, as it gently drains water from the tissue.

Rosemary also helps the skin to regenerate after pregnancy.

Environmental influences and the use of improper skin-care products and aggressive cleansing products are also contributing factors. But the good news is that the full spectrum of the healing powers of aromatherapy oils can be brought to bear where skin problems are concerned. There are essential oils that encourage healthy cell growth, improve circulation, detoxify the body, and help to reduce itchiness and pain.

For skin problems as well as other disorders, this rule always applies: Choose those oils that you like best, and use them to create the appropriate room climate. Inhaling from the scent bottle also works well. However, it's important to note that care should be taken with certain essential oils that can irritate the skin, even if they are heavily diluted.

Healing Wounds and Alleviating Pain

Animals in the wild try to heal themselves if they are ill, injured, or in pain by eating certain healing plants. Humans in ancient times probably observed them doing this and then imitated their behavior. Because the ingestion of essential oils is controversial, I suggest instead to flavor your food with plenty of the respective herbs. Not only will your food taste great, but the herbs will also aid the healing process. If you are unable to obtain fresh herbs, such as rosemary, marjoram, basil, or tarragon, see if you can buy herbs that are preserved in oil. Spices, like nutmeg, ginger, and cinnamon, can be used, in small doses, to treat illnesses that would react to their corresponding oils. In addition, herbal teas, such as chamomile, fennel, anise, and peppermint, or teas containing mixtures of such herbs foster a speedier recovery.

The Most Effective Aroma Oils for Wounds and Pain

SORE ABDOMEN

Apply warm compresses or massages with anise, fennel, chamomile, and/or lavender. Drink hot wormwood tea.

PAINFUL TONSILS

Inhale frequently with benzoin, lavender, or thyme. Also, take a lot of vitamin C, preferably through fresh citrus fruit and juices and green salads.

BURNS

Apply diluted lavender, cajeput, chamomile, myrtle, or niaouli oil.

ACHING MUSCLES

If muscles are tense, take hot baths or apply compresses and rubs with jasmine, chamomile, lavender, clary sage, or juniper. After overexertion, use chamomile, lavender, marjoram, or rosemary.

BACK PAIN

Hot baths and massages with ginger, lavender, marjoram, pepper, or rosemary oil are useful if the pain is due to tension or physical or mental exertion. In the case of an injury or a dislocation of a bone or a joint,

the above treatment will support the treatment of a chiropractor or a doctor.

SORE THROAT

Gargle repeatedly with 1 drop of thyme in a glass of water. You can also use ginger or lemon. Inhale with lavender or benzoin.

NEURALGIA

Apply hot compresses with cajeput, geranium, chamomile, lavender, marjoram, clary sage, or rosemary. Try out different oils until you find the one that is most effective for you.

CUTS OR SIMILAR WOUNDS

For small wounds, dab on some undiluted lavender, chamomile, niaouli, yarrow, or tea tree oil. For larger wounds, apply hot compresses with one or several of the above oils. If the wound is healing poorly, apply compresses with bergamot, myrrh, or tea tree.

HEADACHES

Rub diluted peppermint oil onto your forehead, temples, and neck. Diluted eucalyptus, lavender, rose-

mary, sage, and lemon oil are also suitable. If the headache persists, apply cold compresses with one of these oils.

EARACHE

In light cases, soak a swab of cotton in lavender, and carefully insert it into your ear. Alternatively, blend 1 teaspoon of almond or olive oil with 3 drops of lavender, chamomile, or niaouli, and drip some into your ear. In severe cases, always consult a doctor.

TOOTHACHE

As a first-aid measure, dab a cotton ball soaked in clove oil onto the affected tooth and gums. Put a hot compress with a few drops of chamomile on your cheek. If the gums are inflamed, dab the affected part with orange, rose, or cypress.

SORE STOMACH

Cold compresses and/or rubs with basil, fennel, chamomile, peppermint, tea tree, or cinnamon. If the pain is accompanied by nausea, basil and peppermint are preferable.

Widely cultivated for its aromatic leaves and spikes of purple flowers, lavender is often used in sachets. The oil, when used in baths and massages, is helpful in relieving the pain of rheumatism. In baths, it can also help to reduce or even eliminate headaches.

If one organ is diseased, a person's organism as a whole will suffer. Aromatherapy oils affect not only the afflicted parts but also the entire organism.

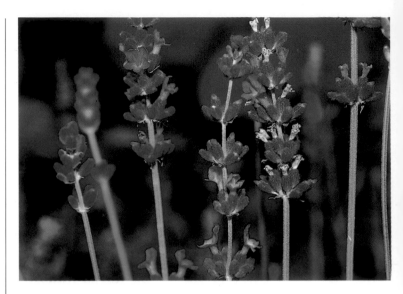

Lavender—the Best-Known Healing Oil

Lavender oil contains more than 260 active ingredients—this explains the oil's versatility. Its pain-relieving and antiseptic properties are useful in treating burns or other wounds, abscesses, eczema, ulcers, and insect bites, whereas its antispasmodic effect helps in relieving a stiff neck, headaches, earaches, neuralgia, and aching muscles. Those suffering from rheumatism or sciatica problems will also benefit from a massage or a hot bath containing lavender. Furthermore, lavender oil improves circulation if applied to dry skin.

Infectious Diseases

An infectious disease is a disease that is caused by viruses and bacteria entering the body and growing and multiplying there. In the case of colds and similar complaints, the pathogens are usually transmitted through sneezing, coughing, or skin contact. Lyme disease, however, is transmitted through tick bites.

Essential oils have proven to be beneficial in treating infections. Garlic, lavender, clove, sage, and thyme prevent bacteria from multiplying, whereas bergamot, eucalyptus, and, most of all, tea tree are effective in fighting viruses. The body's own defenses are strengthened by using angelica, bergamot, eucalyptus, lavender, niaouli, rosemary, and, again, tea tree. These oils can also drastically reduce the risk of infection.

Where infectious diseases are concerned, you should always consult a doctor. However, aromatherapy can be used as an adjunct to a doctor's treatment, alleviating discomfort and accelerating the healing process. Conventional medicines and essential oils are compatible, and one type of treatment doesn't impair the effects of the other.

Specific Blends for Enhanced Effectiveness

One of the interesting properties of essential oils is that, if they are blended with one another, their effectiveness is increased; it's as if they want to spur each other on to do the best they can. We can make use of this property by taking our preferred aroma oil and adding small amounts of any of the other healing oils to it. If you have a cold, you can use tea tree oil as the main oil and add fir, myrtle, and cajeput. Similarly, eucalyptus could be used as the main oil and be supplemented with myrrh, niaouli, and tea tree.

Bronchitis

Bronchitis is an inflammation of the respiratory organs. It usually starts with a dry, painful cough, and it is at this stage that treatment is most effective. Inhaling with chamomile and thyme alleviates pain and reduces the tickling in the throat.

Aroma oils lend themselves to being used in conjunction with other natural remedies. Bronchitis responds well to marshmallow tea, which is prepared cold and left to infuse for two hours. Lime-blossom tea has expectorant properties, so it 's good to drink if you have a cold. Elder-flower tea will cause you to sweat if you have a fever, and gargling with sage and drinking arnica tea relieve a sore throat.

Eucalyptus oil has the most significant effect on the respiratory tract. As an essential oil, as tea, or for inhalation, it has expectorant and anti-inflammatory properties, and also lowers fever and kills germs.

Marjoram oil has expectorant and antispasmodic properties, and is therefore beneficial in treating coughs, hoarseness, and inflammation of the throat. Its warming effect makes it useful when recovering from a cold, and it also has a relaxing and calming effect.

Colds

We often get colds in the fall and the winter as an unwelcome consequence of cold and wet weather. Colds cause noses and eyes to run and throats to become raw and sore. With infections of this kind that haven't yet developed into full-blown influenza, bronchitis, or tonsillitis, immediate treatment with tea tree and eucalyptus oil is advisable. Add 3 to 5 drops of these oils to a handkerchief, and inhale several times a day. You can also add these oils to your essence burner. A warm bath with a few drops of these oils will help as well, but be sure to go to bed afterward and to wrap up warmly.

The Flu

The flu is the next step up from a common cold. It is usually accompanied by a high temperature, a headache, and aching limbs, and can last as long as a week. The flu shouldn't be treated lightly, and you need to get enough rest afterward to avoid a relapse. Tea tree oil is helpful when you have the flu, as is marjoram oil.

Inflammation of the Throat

Throat inflammation usually occurs when there is a bacterial infection of the throat's lining. In more serious cases, the infection attacks the tonsils as well and develops into tonsillitis. If the body's defenses are weakened, pathogens can enter the throat by way of the mouth and cause the inflammation. Eucalyptus, chamomile, lavender, oregano, and tea tree are all anti-inflammatory and pain-reducing oils.

When Not to Use Aroma Oils

❧ If you are using the emergency drops of Bach's flower remedies, you must not use aromatherapy oils at the same time.

❧ Homeopathic medicines are incompatible with essential oils, as they reduce each other's effectiveness.

The Internal Organs

When used in creating the correct room climate, or in baths, rubs, and compresses, or when inhaled directly from the scent bottle, essential oils can also influence disorders of the internal organs. The healing ingredients of the essential oils travel by way of the respiratory system or through the pores of the skin to the affected parts.

The Bladder

Painful bladder complaints are best treated with bergamot added to baths and chamomile and lavender in rubs. Sandalwood presents a good alternative. You could also consider cajeput, fennel, myrtle, juniper, cedar, and cinnamon. Hot compresses with chamomile bring extra pain relief, and it's also a good idea to drink lots of hot chamomile tea.

The Gallbladder

Pain relief for gallstones can be achieved with gentle rubs using lavender, rose, and rosemary. If the gallbladder is inflamed, rosemary is the best option. Immortelle and parsley provide relief as well. A bilious colic can be com-

The anti-inflammatory properties of chamomile are helpful in alleviating bladder complaints. Chamomile also has diuretic and antispasmodic effects, and, when used in steam hip baths (see below), kills germs and improves circulation.

REMEDY

STEAM HIP BATH

Add 3 drops of chamomile blue, 3 drops of melissa 30 percent or 1 drop of melissa 100 percent or lavender to 1 to 2 quarts, or liters, of hot water.

The body adjusts to long-term illnesses. Therefore, try to overcome such illnesses very gently, as opposed to taking drastic measures.

Camphor, garlic, lavender, peppermint, neroli, rose, rosemary, and ylang-ylang are all cardiotonic oils. Rosemary tea (1 teaspoon of the dried herb per cup) has a stimulating effect on circulation and on a weak heart.

Immortelle essence is obtained from the plant's golden-yellow flowers. The oil has antibacterial, antiviral, and anti-inflammatory properties. It improves lymphatic drainage and activates liver function, so that toxins are flushed out of the system more effectively. In order to activate and strengthen the liver, it's advisable to take 1 drop of immortelle essence twice daily. In addition, warm compresses with equal parts of immortelle and rosemary are beneficial.

bated with hot compresses of chamomile, melissa, and/or yarrow.

The Heart

If you frequently suffer from palpitations, or tachycardia, take daily baths with lavender, neroli, rose, and/or ylang-ylang, and rub your chest with the respective massage oil. In addition, it's advisable to ingest a lot of garlic oil, preferably in the form of (virtually) odor-free capsules, or to eat a lot of fresh garlic. Cardiac arrhythmia will disappear with the regular use of chamomile, neroli, peppermint, rose, and/or rosemary in rubs and added to baths.

The Larynx

If your larynx is inflamed, it's advisable to frequently inhale benzoin, lavender, myrtle, sandalwood, and/or thyme. If you lose your voice due to laryngitis, rubbing your neck all over with sandalwood oil will help. Thyme, lemon, or cypress are also suitable.

The Liver

Many demands are put on the liver, and, to support it in breaking down toxins, baths with immortelle, chamomile, peppermint, rosemary, juniper, and lemon are helpful. Applying warm (never hot) compresses with one or more of the above oils relieves acute problems, whereas compresses with rose oil are best for those who have had one drink too many. It's recommended to treat cirrhosis of the liver with lemon oil.

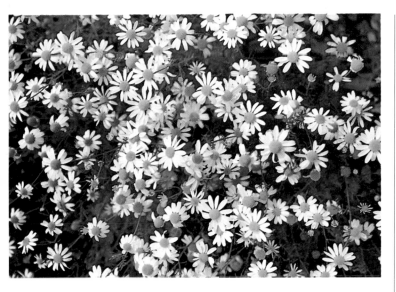

Chamomile oil is called "liquid gold" and is very expensive. However, because of its healing effect on the skin and its balancing effect on the psyche, it should be part of your essential oils home medicine cabinet.

TIP
Juniper, rosemary, fennel, thyme, and peppermint will help relieve nausea and a headache after a night of heavy drinking.

The Stomach

If you have a sore stomach, you will find cold compresses and rubs with anise, tarragon, fennel, geranium, peppermint, or sandalwood very soothing. To relieve stomach cramps, basil, chamomile, clary sage, melissa, and/or tea tree oil are recommended. Stomach ulcers are generally best treated with basil, cajeput, chamomile, peppermint, or lemon.

The Kidneys

If the function of the kidneys is impaired, they can be strengthened with baths and rubs using orange, sandalwood, and yarrow. A doctor's treatment of inflammation of the kidneys, or of pyelitis, can be supplemented with eucalyptus, chamomile, melissa, yarrow, or cypress, or with fir, sandalwood, and juniper. If the patient is in acute pain, inhaling the scent directly from the bottle will bring immediate relief; then the patient should continue with baths and rubs.

Eucalyptus, fennel, rosemary, sage, and thyme are all diuretics. Due to its antispasmodic, anti-inflammatory, and blood-cleansing properties, yarrow oil can also be used to treat kidney complaints. Use it in compresses, ointments, baths, and bandages.

Garlic dilates blood vessels, lowers blood pressure, and has stimulating and antispasmodic properties. Its exceptional healing powers strengthen the body's defenses; therefore, garlic can be said to improve our overall health and help prevent immune deficiencies.

A room scented with benzoin, jasmine, chamomile, rose, sandalwood, and ylang-ylang can do a lot for a cancer patient's comfort and sense of well-being.

Cancer

No one as yet can claim a cure for cancer, aromatherapists included, of course. One of the theories about this terrible disease is that an immune deficiency may be partly responsible. This has by no means been proven, but there is no doubt that it is highly advisable to do everything you can to strengthen the immune system when you are suffering from such a serious disease.

A number of essential oils are suitable, including bergamot, tarragon, eucalyptus, geranium, garlic, clove, sage, cedar, cypress, and onion. It's also interesting to note that garlic and onions, when eaten fresh, play an important role in the treatment of cancer in alternative medicine.

Gentle Massages

British hospitals reflect an open-minded attitude toward aromatherapy, and often include regular gentle massages with essential oils in their treatment of cancer patients. These massages improve the patient's overall sense of well-being and help combat acute pain. In Norway, it is common to apply some lavender oil after radiation treatment, to prevent damage from radiation and limit the damage that has already taken place.

Emotional Climate and Room Climate

Depression and fears often plague cancer patients more than other people who are seriously ill. Foremost are the fears of a long and painful death, and of what can be expected after death. These fears can be overcome with the help of aromatherapy, or at least lessened.

Rose Oil for the Dying

❧ Real rose oil, although quite expensive, is very well suited to helping a dying person move on. It has a calming and mood-lifting effect, chases away depression, and creates an atmosphere of love and care that helps to lessen even the worst pain.

❧ Mix 1 drop of rose oil with a little pure alcohol and distilled water. The concentration is determined by the amount of water added, and the rose scent should always pervade strongly. Spray this mixture into the room, and pour some into a scent bottle.

You can do a lot for someone who is terminally ill by showing him or her your respect and affection. Essential oils can help to let emotions come to the surface.

Dizziness, Faintness, and Shock

In the olden days, if a lady fainted, she was often revived with the help of a little bottle, which probably contained camphor. Camphor activates the circulation and strengthens the heart and the nerves. It can also help a person to overcome depression and to think more clearly.

Inhaling from the Bottle

Neroli and peppermint can also be used to revive someone who has fainted, as can ginger, lavender, and rosemary. Breathe in the scent, and rub a drop into each temple, undiluted for once. Neroli can help to allay fear, whereas peppermint is stimulating and antispasmodic. On awakening, it's best to drink a cup of hot peppermint tea with honey.

If you are prone to dizziness, always carry a small bottle with either basil, lavender, peppermint, rosemary, or thyme, and use it as soon as you feel a spell coming on.

The flowers of the bitter orange tree have a sweet scent, which stimulates the heart and circulation. The scent is named after a 16th-century princess: Neroli. It also has a calming, relaxing, and harmonizing effect. The best way to achieve this is to add 1 to 2 drops of neroli to a teaspoon of honey and then dissolve this mixture in half a cup of water; take two to three times daily.

The fresh, lemon-like scent of melissa strengthens both the body and the soul. It lowers the blood pressure and the heart rate, and it is calming and soothes overwrought nerves.

Scenting Rooms

If you get dizzy at night when you turn over in your bed, scent your bedroom and your pillow as a precautionary measure and have your scent bottle handy on your bedside table. For someone who has suffered a shock, quiet and warmth are paramount. It's best to lie down if possible and cover up.

The scents of neroli and peppermint oil are the most effective, but chamomile, lavender, melissa, and petitgrain are very useful too; inhale directly from the scent bottle, and scent the room as well.

Minor Complaints

Flatulence

REMEDY

WIND-CALMING OIL

Blend 5 drops of anise oil with 1 tablespoon of almond oil; then add 3 drops each of fennel, coriander, and caraway oils. Shake vigorously. Take 2 drops daily on 1 teaspoon of honey before meals.

I recommend taking the Wind-Calming Oil internally (see sidebar). As an alternative, angelica, which is contained in certain liqueurs, may also be taken internally, but only occasionally. Add 2 or 3 drops of the oil to a piece of bread, and chew it before meals. *However, children must not ingest angelica oil!*

Hot compresses with angelica, bergamot, fennel, chamomile, melissa, and/or yarrow will alleviate the pain in a gentler manner than the oral remedies, and are therefore preferred. For children suffering from flatulence, use hot compresses with chamomile oil. All of the above healing oils for this common complaint will also be beneficial when used in an essence burner.

Lumbago

It has been said that lumbago will disappear as suddenly as it appeared. Nevertheless, while you have it, you will want to do something to reduce the pain. Rubs with a massage oil, containing ginger, camphor, peppermint, and/or pepper oil, work well.

Hemorrhoids

Taking hip baths at body temperature (not a hot bath!) and enriched with myrtle, yarrow, and cypress will help a great deal. You can easily make a cream for hemorrhoids yourself by following the formula in the margin.

Corns

The best-known treatment for corns is garlic oil. Apply it undiluted with a cotton swab. As a substitute, you can use fennel, lemon, or onion oil. Apply a Band-Aid afterward to absorb the oil.

Hiccups

If caused by nerves, hiccups can be so persistent and distressing that sufferers will not be able to sleep and, in their despair, will ask to be hospitalized. However, the torment can quickly be brought to an end by taking a lump of sugar with 1 or 2 drops of basil, cumin, dill, tarragon, or caraway oil. Ancient Chinese medicine recommended sandalwood for persistent hiccups.

REMEDY

CREAM FOR HEMORRHOIDS

Add 8 drops each of myrtle and cypress oil to 1.75 ounces, or 50 grams, of naturally pure hamamelis cream. Keep stirring until the oils have been absorbed into the cream. Use regularly.

The sweet scent of sandalwood has been used in ayurvedic medicine for centuries. Its antispasmodic properties help stop hiccups; it also has antiseptic, antiinflammatory, and calming properties.

Scents for Children

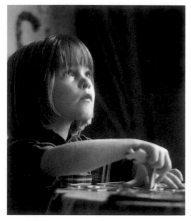

Children naturally enjoy pleasing scents.

From our earliest childhood onward, scents have an important influence on us. We develop something like a "smells register," whereby the memories that are associated with certain smells will be recalled instantly when we come into contact with these smells. It's up to us to encourage the development of the sense of smell in our children, as well as that of all of their senses, so that they will grow up fully enjoying life.

General Benefits

Rosemary has a stimulating effect on the heart and circulation. A few drops on a handkerchief will improve your child's concentration and memory, as well as his or her ability to cope with stress at school.

If a child's room is scented with pleasant aromas, it will convey an atmosphere of security and warmth. Children are especially fond of the scents of benzoin, honey, chamomile, lime, mandarin, neroli, orange, rose, and vanilla. Due to the fire risk, it's best not to use essence burners in a child's room; instead, use an aroma stone or a spray.

Coping with School

In ancient Rome, pupils wore wreaths of rosemary to improve their memory. Just a few drops of rosemary oil will improve concentration tremendously. Therefore, you might want to give your child a handkerchief with a few drops of rosemary on it to take to school. For stress due to exams, the additional use of lavender and ylang-ylang is helpful. Children who are particularly agitated are best calmed down with the scent of clary sage. And a bath before bedtime with a little lavender oil can work wonders.

If a child rejects a certain scent, don't force him or her to put up with it, because the desired effect will certainly not materialize. Rather, choose a different oil that doesn't offend the child's nose. For example, instead of rosemary use basil, or instead of clary sage try lavender or benzoin.

Oils for Timid Children

Timid children react well to benzoin, chamomile, neroli, rose, and vanilla. A nicely scented bath is recommended before bedtime, and the child's room should be scented with a spray or the aroma stone. Gentle massages produce good results too.

Changing Scents in a Child's Room

Children who grow up with essential oils are generally more relaxed, confident, and cheerful than other children. A child's natural desire to explore the world should also be taken into account where aroma oils are concerned. Change the oils in your child's room frequently, and thereby create new stimuli and impulses. But remember to use oils sparingly—do not overdo it.

First Aid for Ear, Nose, and Throat Problems

Nosebleeds

If a child has a nosebleed, soak a small cotton swab in ice-cold water, add a drop of myrrh or lemon oil, and insert it into the affected nostril. The child will have to sit still for a while with his or her head bent forward. If the bleeding doesn't stop, you should consult a doctor.

Change the scents in a child's room every now and then. This way, you will introduce a new stimulus and prevent the child from becoming dependent on a certain scent.

TIP
In the case of a nosebleed, add a drop of myrrh or lemon oil to a cotton swab and insert it into the bleeding nostril.

Complaints of the Respiratory Tract

TIP
During the cold season, always maintain a supply of those oils that have proven most effective with your family in the treatment of colds.

If a child's nose is congested, have the child inhale hot chamomile vapors. Two drops of oil in a bowl of hot water are sufficient. Afterward, wrap the child up warmly in bed. Eucalyptus, pine needle, myrtle, and tea tree are effective oils in fighting colds. Have the child smell the scents from the bottles directly, and spray rooms daily with a blend of all four oils (1 drop of each). During the night, 4 drops on the aroma stone will help induce restful sleep. Coughs can be remedied in the same way, with benzoin, eucalyptus, peppermint (only for children more than six years old), and thyme.

If a child suffers from a sore throat as well, dilute sandalwood oil with some sweet almond oil and rub this into the neck area. Gargling with 1 drop of thyme or lemon added to a glass of warm water will thoroughly disinfect the throat.

Cloves kill germs and act as a strong disinfectant. If you or your child suffers from a toothache, apply some clove oil to the affected tooth or hold a clove against it; then see the dentist.

A Secret Chinese Remedy for Colds

❦ Take a bottle of sandalwood oil or, alternatively, basil, dill, or tarragon.

❦ Close your mouth firmly, and inhale the scent straight from the bottle. This increases the intensity of the scent.

Toothache

A toothache inevitably hits when it is difficult or impossible to get to the dentist-say, late in the evening or on holidays. As a first-aid measure, drip some clove oil onto a cotton ball and press it against the sore tooth. Clove oil not only numbs the pain, but it is also a strong disinfectant. This treatment can be repeated whenever necessary. Warm compresses with a few drops of chamomile applied to the cheek can be very helpful as well. If a baby is in pain when teething, the scents of chamomile and lavender will help to alleviate the pain.

Earache

Who, as a child, hasn't suffered occasionally from an earache? Back then, a little warm oil (normal cooking oil) was regarded as a cure-all. However, in aromatherapy, the treatment is more specific: Barely fill a teaspoon with almond or olive oil, warm it to body temperature in your hand, and then blend it with 3 drops of lavender oil. Drip some into the child's ear, while he or she is lying on the ear that is not affected. Once the pain has subsided somewhat, insert a small cotton swab into the affected ear. Alternatively, warm compresses with chamomile or lavender oil will reduce the pain quickly. In addition, massage a little of these oils gently into the skin around the ear. If the child still suffers from pain in the morning, you will need to consult a doctor.

Gentle Remedies for Stomach and Bowel Complaints

Stomach Pains

Stomach pains are often caused by indigestion. A warm compress with some tarragon, chamomile, lavender, or marjoram oil will produce quick relief. These oils can also be applied by means of massage. If the child feels nauseous at the same time, basil, peppermint (not suitable for

Distraction frequently helps children bear pain more easily. Essential oils can distract children, in that they draw their attention to a pleasant smell sensation.

Warm compresses or gentle massages with tarragon, chamomile, lavender, or marjoram help alleviate stomach pains.

Stomach and bowel problems don't need to be treated with strong medicines right away. Frequently essential oils that are related to herbs and spices will do the job just as well.

Treatment for Intestinal Parasites

❧ Serve the child plenty of fresh garlic and onions- for example, finely chopped on bread, in tomato salads, or in quark (a low-fat soft cheese) as a filling for jacket potatoes. In addition, serve dishes seasoned with caraway and cinnamon.

❧ Add bergamot and lavender oil to the aroma stone in the child's room. Of course, you can also use tea tree oil.

❧ Also, give the child lots of fennel and chamomile tea to drink.

❧ Once the parasites have passed and the child's complaints have subsided, it's advisable to repeat the treatment after five to seven days.

children under the age of six), or sandalwood will help. The child should inhale the scent straight from the bottle, or it can be used in a spray or on the aroma stone.

Wormwood tea is a real miracle cure for such cases, but unfortunately it is so bitter that it probably won't be very appealing to a child, even if you add honey to it. However, good results have also been achieved with fennel, chamomile, and peppermint tea. These teas encourage the production of digestive juices and have a calming effect on stomach and bowel cramps.

Constipation

Children often suffer from constipation when they are on a holiday or in a new environment. This can easily be treated with aromatherapy remedies.

As a rule, children rarely suffer from constipation, because they generally get plenty of exercise and eat a balanced diet. Therefore, constipation in children is usually seen as a sign of some kind of stress, or as a consequence of fear, shock, or problems that have not been dealt with. Gentle, clockwise massages of the tummy with a little marjoram, rosemary, or fennel oil, diluted with jojoba oil, will encourage bowel function.

As far as daily meals are concerned, it's important for the child to eat a lot of fruit and vegetables, and to drink fruit juices and several cups of fennel tea a day. If these measures don't produce any results, then underlying emotional problems may be the cause and perhaps a therapist should be consulted.

Diarrhea

Chamomile, neroli, sandalwood, and cypress are very effective oils in the treatment of diarrhea. Gently rub them onto the sore tummy, and also let the child inhale the scents straight from the bottle. Use the scents that the child likes best. In addition, give the child plenty of luke-warm peppermint tea to drink, sweetened with sugar (never give milk), and when the appetite returns, offer some pretzel sticks or some melba toast. The child will need to be wrapped up warmly.

Treating Minor Injuries and Bruises

The following suggestions for treatment apply to adults as well as to children. The reason they appear in this chapter is because children get bruises repeatedly.

❧ Burns and Minor Grazes

Dab a few drops of undiluted lavender or tea tree oil onto the wound immediately. In the case of burns, lavender, in particular, prevents tissue from swelling and blisters from forming. When the pain-reducing effect of the oil dies down, the treatment can safely be repeated.

Cypress oil has a warm, spicy scent, and anti-spasmodic and antiseptic properties. It is obtained from the needle-like leaves and the twigs of the evergreen cypress tree.

In the case of burns and scalds, lavender relieves pain immediately and prevents swelling and the formation of blisters. Its calming effect also helps alleviate shock, which often accompanies burns and scalds. As a first-aid measure, remove any clothing covering the burnt areas, and then cool the burn under running water; after that, apply lavender oil to the burn until the pain lets up.

Where grazes are concerned, the disinfectant effect of tea tree oil is beneficial. For grazes, dab a few drops of the pure oil onto the cleansed wound.

❦ Sprained Ankle

Cold compresses with lavender, chamomile, peppermint, and tea tree oil are best for swelling and bruising. Afterward, a doctor should bandage the ankle.

❦ Bruises

Apply cold compresses. Fennel and lavender have proven to be particularly effective. Once the bruises turn a greenish-yellow color, rub on some undiluted rosemary oil so that they will heal faster.

Essential Oils and Childhood Diseases

Where serious illnesses are concerned, essential oils are no substitute for treatment from a doctor, but they can support the treatment, alleviate complaints, accelerate recovery, and strengthen the child's natural defenses.

If you suspect that a child has broken a bone, go to see a doctor immediately. Broken bones have to be set correctly, so that they won't grow together in the wrong position.

Being ill is a major experience for a child, and you can help a child to cope with it in a positive manner.

If Your Child Wets the Bed	
1 Before bedtime, give your child a bath with 2 drops of juniper oil and 1 drop each of bergamot and cypress.	the juniper scent straight from the bottle. **3** Continue this treatment for two to three weeks.
2 Also, add 1 drop of each oil to the aroma stone, and let your child inhale	**4** If the problem persists, consider consulting a therapist.

Essential Oils for the Most Common Childhood Diseases

DISEASE	ESSENTIAL OIL
Chicken pox	Cajeput, myrtle, tea tree
Diphtheria	Bergamot
Measles	Bergamot, cajeput, lavender
Scarlet fever	Eucalyptus, myrtle, tea tree
Tonsillitis	Benzoin, lavender, thyme
Whooping cough	Basil, myrtle, thyme

TIP
Spray the child's room with these oils, add a few drops to the aroma stone, and occasionally let your child smell them directly from the bottle.

Disinfecting

The best way to disinfect the air in a child's room and in other rooms is to use tea tree oil or lemon oil. Both oils effectively fight bacteria as well as fungi and viruses. They also reduce the risk of infection. Eucalyptus, peppermint (only suitable for children over the age of six), myrtle, rosemary, and thyme are good for disinfecting rooms, too, and can be used in sprays, in the essence burner, or on the aroma stone. Water used for washing hands can be disinfected with myrtle, sage, or lemon.

Protecting the Immune System

Angelica, bergamot, cajeput, eucalyptus, tea tree, and thyme can be used to protect and strengthen the immune system. To stimulate the appetite once the worst of the illness is over, baths with bergamot, ginger, chamomile, caraway, and lemon have shown good results. Let the child also smell these oils half an hour before mealtimes.

Angelica strengthens the body's defenses, and has a restoring and motivating effect on the body. The oil is obtained from the roots of this robust plant, which can grow higher than 6 feet tall. The aroma is spicy and blends well with citrus scents.

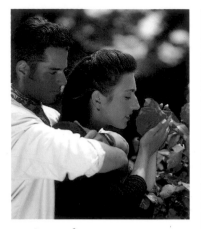

*Certain fragrances can create a
tender, loving atmosphere.*

TIP
*If you have drunk alcohol or
if you are epileptic, avoid
undiluted clary sage.*

**The following oils have
an aphrodisiac effect:
cardamom, cinnamon
geranium, jasmine,
mimosa, rose, sandal-
wood, tonka bean,
tuberose, vanilla, vet-
iver, and ylang-ylang.**

Scents for Lovers

Scents affect the subconscious relationship between partners, but nevertheless in a very important manner, which
is one of the reasons why the perfume industry is so successful. With the scents that we choose, we influence how
others subconsciously perceive us, and project certain
personality types, such as the sensual, sexually oriented
type, or the rather lively, natural type.

Scents can also influence the atmosphere of a room: A
seducing room spray, along with the right essential oils
added to the essence burner, can easily create a relaxed
and loving or erotic atmosphere. Candlelight will enhance
the romantic ambience, as will wine and some gentle
music. However, stay away from scented and colored
lamp oils. They look very pretty, but unfortunately are
highly toxic.

Arousing Tender Emotions

Herbalists of old knew how to mix aphrodisiac lotions
and potions, which the object of one's desire couldn't
resist. Although fail-safe formulas are few and far
between these days, several essential oils can create a
magic atmosphere and encourage secret desires. First of
all, it's important to forget about everyday troubles.
Benzoin, clary sage, neroli, patchouli, rose, and ylang-
ylang are some of the scents that will help you and your
partner to relax.

Experiment to find out which blends used in your
essence burner capture you and your partner the most. If

possible, try adopting your partner's favorite oil as your own and using it in your perfume (see "Tips for the Correct Use of Aroma Oils") and other cosmetics. But remember that we get used to even the most exciting scents after a while. If you want to keep the electricity flowing between you and your lover, it's a good idea to change your chosen scents every now and then.

Seducing with Scents

A woman can signal her erotic interest best with jasmine, whereas a man should use sandalwood. With these oils, it will be difficult for your partner to remain cool and calm. However, don't use too much—less can often be more. Your perfume or facial toner should not be overpowering, but subtle and suggestive.

Rose oil, alone or used in blends, will give the female longing for closeness a soft, loving note. Ylang-ylang is best suited to vivacious women who send out strongly erotic vibes. Just a touch will be enough.

The Female Oils—The Male Oils

Female	Oils	Male	Oils
Angelica	Iris	Ambrette seed	Mimosa
Benzoin	Jasmine	Basil	Myrrh
Cinnamon rose	Lavender	Caraway seed	Narcissus
Chamomile	Lime	Cardamom	Orange
Coriander	Mimosa	Cedar	Palmarosa
Cypress	Neroli	Cinnamon	Pine
Fennel	Rose	Ginger	Rosewood
Grapefruit	Rosemary	Lemon	Sandalwood
Hyacinth	Tuberose	Melissa	Vetiver
	Ylang-ylang		

Rosewood oil is another aphrodisiac. It is obtained from the rosewood tree, which is indigenous to the tropics and under threat from extinction due to the clearing of the rain forest. Although rosewood oil is for sale, for environmental reasons we should think twice before buying it.

Ylang-ylang means "flower of flowers" in Malay. The tree, with its large flowers, exudes an erotic scent, which actually stimulates the pituitary gland, which in turn releases endorphins. These endorphins create a state of euphoria, increase desire, and encourage us to let our emotions flow freely.

Ylang-ylang can also release tension and inhibitions in women who have trouble feeling relaxed and carefree. Perfumes with benzoin, hyacinth, and iris, and a dash of lime, cinnamon rose, and tuberose, are very sensuous. Geranium has a stimulating effect on both men and women; cumin and ambrette seed oil are even more stimulating.

Cedar, on the other hand, is a typically male scent, which women love. Its rugged character can be softened and made more intimate by adding clary sage and orange. Other harmonious scent blends are sandalwood with cumin, and lime with geranium. A hint of ambrette seed or vetiver will increase the effect.

Awakening Suppressed Feelings

In matters of love, you can't force anything— you can only support that which wants to come forth. The aphrodisiac scents of vanilla, cinnamon, labdanum, and rose may be able to help in this respect.

Introverted people tend to react to the warm and comforting scents of vanilla or cinnamon oil. Adding a little patchouli or vetiver to them in the essence burner will give the scent a certain edge. Labdanum and rose are also well suited to "late starters."

The harmonizing effects of geranium and clary sage can help to ease emotional strains within a relationship. Honey oil, too, can help to reduce tension between partners. Honey oil is best blended with hyacinth, jasmine, rose, vetiver, and/or ylang-ylang.

Hyacinth, cinnamon rose, and tuberose have a strongly erotic effect. They can also help people who harbor feelings of distrust and have inhibitions, bringing out in them the feeling that life is worth living, and that love isn't just something that happens to other people.

If you have fears regarding a new affair, because you have been deeply hurt in a previous relationship, peru balsam, tonka bean, and vanilla will have beneficial effects.

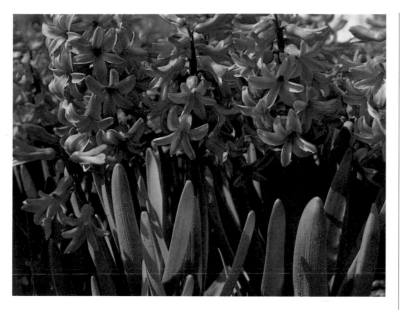

The intoxicating scent of hyacinths opens the heart and allows dormant feelings to blossom. Hyacinth is therefore the essential oil that is generally the best suited to lovers.

Overcoming Impotence and Frigidity

Emotional problems and stress can lead to frigidity in women and impotence in men. However, if the cause of these problems is having an insensitive, unsympathetic partner, then essential oils will not be able to remedy the situation. Partners have to be open toward each other, and show understanding, if they want to reach sexual harmony again.

Interestingly enough, many of the same oils can have the desired effect on both men and women. Of course, it always depends on the type of person. Iris, jasmine, rose, neroli, and ylang-ylang are considered particularly female oils. Some women, however, react more strongly to typically male scents, such as ginger, cardamom, caraway, and sandalwood. The same holds true for men. You will have to experiment a little, to discover which oils affect both you and your partner the most.

In Asian cultures, jasmine is revered as a symbol of sensual love. It is called "moonlight in the grove" or "queen of the night"—names that bear testimony to its seductive powers. Jasmine can be used as an aroma oil on its own, or as an additive to baths or massage oils.

Savory thyme has been known to increase the libido since ancient times.

Valerian soothes frayed nerves and creates the calm necessary to consider a problem and find a suitable solution.

How to Break Down Barriers in Your Sex Life

❦ Massage each other with a massage oil that you have blended yourselves (see "Tips for the Correct Use Of Aroma Oils"), using one or more of the oils mentioned above. Concentrate the massage on the back and the sacrum.

❦ Take a bath before intercourse (together is best). Add 7 drops each of caraway, geranium, and clary sage to 2 tablespoons of carrier oil, and then add this to the bath water.

❦ Scent your rooms or even your bed linen with aphrodisiac oils, to create a harmonious, sensual atmosphere.

Keeping Jealousy in Check

There are basically two types of jealous people: those who almost explode with anger, and those who usually keep their feelings to themselves and feel extremely sad, while their emotions are eating them up inside.

People in the first category need something to calm them down. Valerian is a good choice, as it sedates slightly, but at the same time cools one down enough to reconsider the situation. Valerian oil can be taken internally, dripped on a lump of sugar. What is even more effective is adding a few drops of valerian to a glass of hot honey water. Geranium, chamomile, peru balsam, rose, and tuberose are also recommended, whether used in the essence burner, in baths, or in cosmetics.

For those who bear their jealousy quietly and suffer inwardly, angelica, bergamot, honey oil, jasmine, peru balsam, rose, and ylang-ylang are the oils that work best.

However, don't expect any miracles in either case, and don't rely on the effects of the essential oils alone. It is crucial that you take time to discuss the issue openly with your partner.

Essential Oils and Sexually Transmitted Diseases

If you have been infected with a sexually transmitted disease, you must see your doctor and undergo treatment not only for yourself but also to prevent the disease from spreading. However, essential oils can be used to support and supplement the doctor's treatment.

With syphilis, washes or cold compresses with sassafras or lemon support medical treatment. With gonorrhea, benzoin, bergamot, cajeput, lavender, and sandalwood can be used in addition to the above two oils. Eating lots of garlic (fresh or in capsules) will help to strengthen the body's defenses.

CAUTION!
Essential oils must not come in contact with condoms.

Frequent washes with sassafras, lemon, benzoin, bergamot, cajeput, lavender, and sandalwood help in the treatment of sexually transmitted diseases due to their antibacterial and disinfectant properties.

Oils That Can Be Used to Protect Yourself

ESSENTIAL OIL	EFFECT
Bergamot	Antibacterial, disinfectant
Cinnamon	Antiviral, antibacterial, disinfectant
Oregano	Antiviral, antibacterial, antifungal
Palmarosa	Antiviral, antibacterial
Peru balsam	Antibacterial, disinfectant
Tea tree	Antiviral, antibacterial, antifungal, detoxifying
Thyme	Antiviral, antibacterial, antifungal

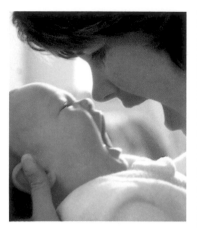

Aromatherapy can be beneficial for mothers of young infants.

During pregnancy, avoid baths and massages with the following essential oils: basil, cinnamon, clary sage, coriander, dill, hyssop, juniper, marjoram, myrrh, sage, and thyme. During the first four months of pregnancy, also avoid fennel, peppermint, rose, and rosemary.

Scents for Women

Essential Oils for Pregnant Women

A woman expecting a child will best be able to cope with the accompanying emotional and physical strains if she is in a harmonious and relaxed atmosphere. It's important for her to be able to fully enjoy the anticipation of the new life growing inside her, and aromatherapy can help bring out these positive feelings.

Seeing, Hearing, and Smelling Beautiful Things

Everything that is pleasant for the eyes, ears, and nose will contribute to a good-natured disposition, will reinforce other positive influences, and can have a beneficial effect on the fetus. It has been suggested that fetuses that have experienced the effects of essential oils indirectly in their mother's womb develop into calmer and more balanced babies.

There are, however, some essential oils that should be avoided by pregnant women, because they can cause a miscarriage. If you are expecting a child, refrain from baths and massages with basil, cinnamon, clary sage, coriander, dill, hyssop, juniper, marjoram, myrrh, sage, and thyme. All other scents can be safely enjoyed.

In Preparation for the Birth

One week before the estimated date of birth, you can start with gentle massages of the back and the stomach, using jasmine or lavender oil. This relaxes the muscles and helps them to prepare for labor. From the same time onward, it's also advisable to take baths adding 6 drops of either one of these oils.

Pain Relief and Relaxation During the Birth

Jasmine and lavender oil are also very well suited to alleviating pain during the birth. You can blend your own massage oil with them and apply gentle rubs or warm compresses. In addition, jasmine intensifies contractions, thereby shortening labor. Myrrh, clary sage, and sage have the same effect as jasmine. Which you use depends on which scents you prefer.

Mandarin oil will contribute to relaxation, and rosewood reduces stress. Cold compresses with verbena will stimulate the contractions of the uterus.

You can scent the room where the baby will be born with verbena, jasmine, lavender, mandarin, and/or rosewood. Immediately after the birth, a massage with diluted jasmine oil is advisable so that the placenta can be delivered quickly.

Essential Oils to Use After the Birth

Jasmine oil is also very well suited to preventing or treating depression just after childbirth. If you find the scent too overpowering, use lavender, neroli, rose, rosewood, or ylang-ylang instead. Three or four of these oils used in conjunction will reinforce the effects of each one.

Jasmine and lavender relax muscles, thereby helping in preparation for the birth. Their anti-spasmodic and relaxing effects can also make the actual birth easier.

Because the date of the birth cannot be determined exactly, try to prepare well ahead of time, and possibly even give your chosen scent sequence a trial run (it should, of course, contain jasmine).

Stretch marks from pregnancy are best treated with massages using oils that improve circulation and strengthen the connective tissue.

REMEDY

BODY OIL

Add 7 drops of lavender, 3 drops of cedar, 3 drops of sandalwood, 1 drop of rose, and 1 drop of neroli to 100 ml of sweet almond oil or jojoba oil. Gently massage twice daily into the chest, stomach, and hip areas.

If you find that you still haven't conceived after trying for a long time, you should consult your doctor to determine whether or not there are physical causes.

Help for Minor Complaints During Pregnancy

MORNING SICKNESS
Breathe in the scent of peppermint oil.

BACKACHE
Have your back massaged with almond oil to which a few drops of ginger, lavender, and rosemary have been added.

STRETCH MARKS
From the fifth month onward, massage your abdomen and hips with almond oil to which 2 to 3 percent of mandarin or neroli oil have been added.

SWOLLEN LEGS
Massage your legs, always from bottom to top, and use almond or jojoba oil to which a few drops of geranium and rosemary have been added. Put your feet up as often as possible, preferably while you are lying on your back.

Anise, verbena, caraway, and fennel oil, as well as fennel tea, encourage lactation. The essential oils are diluted in carrier oils for this purpose (see "Tips for the Correct Use Of Aroma Oils"), and rubbed on or applied in compresses. Inflamed nipples can be treated in the same way, using geranium, cinnamon rose, and rose. If you are weaning your child off of nursing, apply lukewarm compresses with clary sage, peppermint, and sage.

Why Don't I Conceive?

Some couples desperately long for a child but are unable to conceive. Does the problem lie with him or with her? Accusations and arguments will not resolve the situation; on the contrary, with increasing stress, the chances of conceiving are further reduced. In addition, it is often the strong desire and determination to have a child that prevents women from conceiving.

Baths and Massages to Balance Hormone Levels

If a young woman's periods are irregular or weak, calculating the day of ovulation can turn into a game of luck. Regular baths and massages with geranium or rose will strengthen the uterus and balance hormone levels. Hip baths and/or massages with basil, coriander, thyme, vanilla, hyssop, or cinnamon will encourage the onset of the expected menstruation (therefore, these oils must not be used during pregnancy).

Scents to Help Both Partners Relax

If the cause of the infertility is more of a mental one, relaxing and balancing aroma baths can help both partners. Bergamot, jasmine, clary sage, and neroli are particularly well suited, also combined with rose. Pay attention to the room climate as well, especially in your bedroom, and remember to scent your cosmetics.

Be honest with yourself and your partner: Is there some part of yourself deep inside that doesn't want a baby?

Menstrual Problems

Often the problems start before the actual period has begun. Now commonly called Premenstrual Syndrome (PMS), these problems can appear a few days before menstruation and be emotional as well as physical. Women with PMS often feel bloated, and may experience constipation, headaches, and nausea. On the emotional side, they tend to be overly sensitive, some bursting into tears at the slightest cause, and others exploding with anger at any given moment. Severe depression can occur as well.

REMEDIES

BODY OILS

Add 1 drop of jasmine, 2 drops of clary sage, 3 drops of ylang-ylang, and 5 drops of grapefruit to 700 ml of sweet almond oil and 30 ml of St. John's Wort oil; shake well. Or, add 3 drops of ylang-ylang, 1 drop of rose, 1 drop of cedar, 1 drop of rosemary, and 1 drop of cinnamon rose to 100 ml of sweet almond oil or jojoba oil, and shake well.

Warm compresses applied to the abdomen are relaxing and cause cramps to subside.

How to Control Your Periods

❦ HEAVY AND NORMAL PERIODS

Gentle massages of the abdomen and/or back, using chamomile, lavender, marjoram, and rose.

❦ IRREGULAR PERIODS

Baths, hip baths, rubs, and compresses, with basil, fennel, rosemary, yarrow, juniper, vanilla, or vetiver oil, before the onset of the period.

❦ WEAK PERIODS

Compresses and rubs with the above oils, and also with thyme, but during the period. Relaxation exercises are helpful too.

Overcoming Depression

Ridding the body of excess water can do wonders for alleviating depression and that bloated feeling. Use geranium and rosemary oil to drain the water that has accumulated in the body; this should be done about two to three days before the problem usually appears.

Baths with bergamot, chamomile, rose, and tonka bean, along with scenting the room with the corresponding scent, will also help overcome depression and irritability. Neroli and ylang-ylang have a similarly beneficial effect.

Alleviating Pain

Menstrual pains are best counteracted by gently rubbing on a massage oil containing chamomile, melissa, peppermint, rosemary, and/or tea tree. Warm compresses with one or more of these oils will also bring relief. Try them out to see what is most pleasant for you. A light diet, high in fiber (plenty of fruit, vegetables, and whole-grain cereal products), and avoiding caffeine, alcohol, and nicotine as much as possible, will enhance the positive impact of the oils. Should you experience problems with digestion, however, evening primrose oil will help.

Women's Disorders

It goes without saying that all serious illnesses have to be treated by a doctor or a qualified practitioner of alternative medicine. However, essential oils can play an important role in supporting and supplementing medical treatment.

❧ Vaginal Discharge

There can be several causes of vaginal discharge (see also "Thrush" and "Leukorrhea," below), so it's important to first obtain an exact diagnosis from your doctor. Aromatherapy has achieved very good results with vaginal douches (rubber douches are available at your drugstore). To half a quart, or liter, of boiled water, add 1 teaspoon of pure alcohol that has been blended with 2 to 5 drops of essential oils (see "Thrush" and "Leukorrhea" for specific oils). Shake well and use at body temperature.

❧ Breast Cancer

Never use clary sage, star anise, or cypress (see "Cancer," on page 36).

❧ Uterine Complaints

Use warm compresses, baths, and hip baths with jasmine, melissa, and rose.

❧ Thrush

This is a fungal infection of the vaginal lining. The symptoms are a white discharge, itchiness, and sometimes pain. Use vaginal douches (see "Vaginal Discharge," above) or

TIP
Use your oils sparingly and carefully to avoid unnecessary irritation of the sensitive vaginal lining.

To treat thrush, or itchiness and inflammation in the vagina, prepare a blend of 5 drops of tea tree oil, 5 drops of lavender, 30 ml of St. John's Wort oil, and 20 ml of aloe vera oil. Fill into a glass bottle, shake well, soak a tampon in this blend, and insert the tampon into the vagina.

take hip baths, using tea tree oil. Or, insert tampons soaked in a mixture of pure vegetable oil, such as jojoba or almond, and 2 drops of tea tree oil. For thrush, you can use lavender or myrrh oil as well.

❧ Leukorrhea

As opposed to thrush, this is not a disease. Leukorrhea is a discharge from the vagina due to inflammation or congestion of the mucous membrane. It often occurs in young girls and during the first half of the menstrual cycle, before ovulation. Vaginal douches with bergamot, lavender, myrrh, rosemary, and sandalwood will help.

❧ Inflammation of the Vagina

The symptoms are a yellow-greenish discharge with an unpleasant smell, vaginal swelling, and occasional pain. Vaginal inflammation is usually caused by a fungal infection. Here, the healing powers of yarrow and tea tree used in douches have produced the best results. The effects of these douches will be heightened if you use rosewater as a carrier and blend it with 1 or 2 drops of either of the above oils. Douches with tea tree oil are also suitable. Add 4 to 5 drops of tea tree oil to a cup of warm water, and slowly pour this blend over the genital area. This will help to alleviate itchiness. For a bath, 10 drops of tea tree oil added to hot water are sufficient.

Menopause

During this time in a woman's life, the hormonal balance is disturbed, sometimes causing physical and emotional problems, such as irregular periods (before their complete cessation), breaking out in sweat (hot flashes), depression, troubled sleep, headaches, loss of libido, and sometimes

REMEDY

MENOPAUSE OIL

Blend 3 drops each of geranium, melissa (or fennel), clary sage, and cypress with 20 ml of jojoba oil and half a teaspoon of evening primrose oil. This blend is suitable as a bath oil and a massage oil.

even hair loss. Geranium, melissa, and rose are used for their balancing effect. Clary sage, sage (drinking sage tea is also advisable; pour hot water over finely chopped sage leaves, and infuse for 10 minutes), and cypress are best suited for hot flashes and preventing excessive sweating. Dryness of the vagina, another possible effect of menopause, can be treated with fennel oil (never apply directly!). Ylang-ylang helps counteract loss of libido. However, only treatment of the entire body with massages and baths will bring forth the desired results.

Women going through menopause will find it easier to cope with this notorious midlife crisis and all of its ramifications (including depression) if they use bergamot, jasmine, chamomile, lavender, clary sage, neroli, sandalwood, yarrow, and ylang-ylang. They can be used in baths and massages, as a room spray, in the essence burner, and in cosmetics. (For troubled sleep, refer to the chapter "How to Sleep Like a Baby.")

REMEDY

BATH OIL

Blend 1 drop of jasmine, 1 drop of neroli, 5 drops of sandalwood, 1 drop of styrax, and 1 drop of clary sage with half a cup to a cup of cream, and add to the bath water.

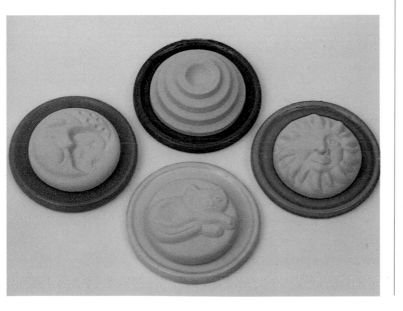

Aroma stones are made from fine fired clay. Their porous texture soaks up the aroma oils and then releases them again very gradually. Lemongrass, geranium, palmarosa, and mint are particularly suited for use with aroma stones.

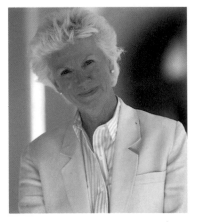

Aromatherapy will keep you young.

Scents for Seniors

Not only can aromatherapy help alleviate the symptoms of many age-related disorders, but it can also assist older people in coping better with the specific issues that arise at this stage. For example, if you have retired recently and are finding everyday existence dreary, the correct essential oils will restore your energy and give you fresh impetus.

Life is worth living at all times and is full of wonders. This message is conveyed by some lovely aroma oils, such as geranium, jasmine, lime, mandarin, rose, ylang-ylang, and lemon. The secret is not to resign yourself to your fate. You can pull yourself up by your own bootstraps, if need be.

Life doesn't have to be dreary! Scents can open you up to new interests and a fresh love of life. Many older people have a rich store of experience that they can draw upon in undertaking new projects. Don't let your abilities go unused!

Loneliness and Despondency

Loneliness is very common in old age, and many people find it difficult to bear. As an antidote to feelings of loneliness, create an environment for yourself that is as pleasant as possible. Set up an essence burner, and add a few drops of fennel, honey, ginger, or chamomile oil to the water. Consciously breathe in the lovely scent, and take time to think about what actions you could take in your life to alleviate your loneliness. Think about meeting new people and, if possible, taking on new projects. Leading an active life is the best way to fight loneliness. Perhaps you could become involved with a charity, or seek out like-minded people, with whom you can go on walks, visit museums, or attend concerts.

Don't allow negative thoughts (for example, I can't do that!) to take hold. Despondency can be treated with ginger, bay, marjoram, rosemary, thyme, and cinnamon. Add 2 or 3 drops of one or two of these oils to your blend in the essence burner. Remember all the things that you can do, and reflect on how many of your abilities are just waiting to be put to good use. Of course, you can achieve something. You can help yourself and help others.

Scents for Gray Days		
Angelica	Cinnamon	Marjoram
Bay	Fennel	Rosemary
Bergamot	Ginger	Thyme
Chamomile	Honey	Ylang-ylang

Memory Lapses and Forgetfulness

A whole score of essential oils is suitable for treating memory lapses and forgetfulness. Basil, peppermint, and rosemary rank first among them. They boost our ability to remember and strengthen our capacity to concentrate.

If you are frequently annoyed over your own forgetfulness, it would be a good idea to always carry a bottle of one of these three essential oils with you. You will have to experiment to determine which of the three oils is most helpful for you. Basil, rosemary, or peppermint? You can also alternate the oils. If used at home in the essence burner, they will help when you are working a crossword puzzle, writing an important letter, compiling the shopping list, or doing other activities that require concentration. As an alternative to these three oils, you can also use eucalyptus, marjoram, clove, hyssop, or stone pine.

Cinnamon oil has a pleasantly warm and sweet scent, which stimulates the heart and circulation. It also creates a cozy, relaxed atmosphere when used in the essence burner or in the bath.

Basil is an excellent essential oil for complaints that occur in old age. Inhale the vapors from the bottle deeply, or take a bath to which a few drops of basil have been added. Basil is especially well suited for treating:

❧ **physical inertia,**
❧ **dizzy spells,**
❧ **mental weakness, and**
❧ **high blood pressure.**

Scents That Improve Memory and Concentration		
Basil	Lemongrass	Petitgrain
Clove	Marjoram	Rosemary
Eucalyptus	Pennyroyal	Savory
Hyssop	Peppermint	Stone pine

If you are desperately looking for your keys, for example, stop and light your essence burner, adding one or more of the above oils, and let the scent take effect for about 10 minutes. Then inhale from the scent bottle. Now when you resume your search, it will be much easier.

Physical Weakness

The oils derived from herbs and spices are the ones that will best treat physical exhaustion. These are savory, ginger, garlic, marjoram, clove, peppermint, rosemary, thyme, juniper, and lemon. These herbs should therefore be used frequently in cooking. Garlic can also be taken in the form of capsules to minimize its unpleasant odor.

Resignation

Once you have overcome physical inertia, it will be easier to deal with resignation, which ultimately stems from a feeling of weakness. Now you need a different set of essential oils. Use geranium, jasmine, lemongrass, mandarin, rose, and ylang-ylang, as well as lemon again, in your essence burner, room spray, baths, and cosmetics. Of course, you can't rely solely on the effects of essential oils. To achieve lasting success, you will also have to maintain a positive attitude and show some initiative.

Bitterness

Anyone who looks back over a fairly long life will not have had only positive experiences in all these years. It's important to realize that you aren't the only one to whom fate has not always been kind. But don't allow yourself to become bitter. Instead, prepare an aroma bath with angelica, honey, jasmine, rose, and/or ylang-ylang (suited for men as well as women). And make plans for an excursion, a visit to the theater, a wander through town—anything that will give you pleasure. Use your inner resources to raise your spirits.

Mental Confusion

Mental confusion can sometimes occur in old age as a consequence of insufficient blood circulation in the brain. In aromatherapy, mental confusion is treated with some of the same essential oils that are used to contend with memory lapses—for example, eucalyptus, peppermint, rosemary, sage, and thyme. Your intellectual abilities will soon improve, because the scents are directly absorbed into the limbic system from the essence burner or the scent bottle.

Thyme is not only an aromatic cooking herb, but it also has exceptional healing powers. If you aren't feeling up to par physically or mentally, the scent of thyme will give you new energy, support you in intellectual endeavors, and improve your concentration. In addition, its antiseptic and germicidal properties are excellent in combating infectious diseases, disorders of the respiratory tract, stomach and bowel complaints, and kidney and bladder problems.

Age-Related Disorders

Gout

Gout is a disturbance of the purine metabolism, and entails deposits of urates in the joints and usually an excessive amount of uric acid in the blood.

Gout can cause inflammations of the joints (see "Healing Physical Complaints"). At first, only one toe or finger segment may be affected. Nevertheless, the attacks are extremely painful. However, cold compresses with benzoin, chamomile, lavender, and rosemary will relieve the pain. In addition, baths and rubs with fennel, juniper, lemon, and cypress will encourage the removal of toxins from the joints. After the heat treatment, you must try to move the affected joint to prevent heat from accumulating, which could aggravate the situation.

Here are some diet tips for gout patients designed to improve their overall condition: Avoid meat, as well as tea, coffee, and alcohol. Eat light meals with lots of fruit and vegetables, and take vitamin A, B, and E supplements if necessary.

REMEDY

BATH OIL FOR URINARY INCONTINENCE

Blend 8 drops of cypress and 3 drops of juniper with 2 tablespoons of almond oil. Add to a hip bath regularly.

Urinary Incontinence or Retention

If you suffer from either of these problems, which despite their wide occurrence are not generally talked about, you will find that aromatherapy can help. Older people cannot always urinate when they want to, and sometimes they urinate involuntarily and uncontrollably, usually in the form of a light dripping. Regular warm (not hot) hip baths with a special blend of essential oils for urinary incontinence will strengthen the muscles of the urinary tract and the bladder.

If you suffer from the opposite problem—hat is, urinary retention—you should use patchouli or juniper oil instead. The way juniper works is a good example of the

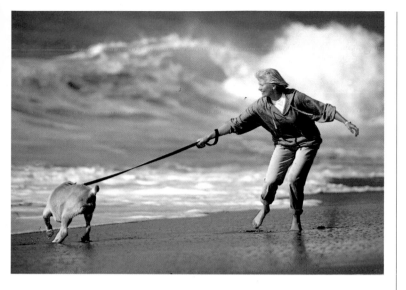

Essential oils can rekindle your love of life, and be a source of physical and mental strength.

balancing effect that many essential oils have: In large amounts, juniper can cause urinary retention; in small doses, it can heal it.

Prostate Problems

With increasing age, the prostate becomes larger, narrowing the urethra as a consequence. Although usually painful, this enlargement is not dangerous, but you should consult your physician nevertheless.

Hip baths with 3 drops each of patchouli, juniper, and onion, added to 2 tablespoons of vegetable oil, can help an enlarged prostate. It's also good to ingest a lot of garlic, also in the form of capsules. Juice made from pumpkin seeds, or a daily dose of 20 to 25 actual seeds, will help as well.

For an inflamed prostate, take baths and hip baths with 4 drops each of fir, juniper, and pine, added to 2 tablespoons of vegetable oil. However, in serious cases, you must consult your doctor.

Juniper oil has stimulating and antispasmodic effects. It disinfects the urinary tract, which is especially beneficial if you suffer from cystitis, urinary calculus, or urinary retention. Furthermore, its spicy, aromatic scent improves circulation and relieves exhaustion.

Varicose Veins and Other Vein Complaints

The best aromatherapy oil for varicose veins and other vein complaints is cypress oil. It should be applied lightly twice daily, diluted with jojoba oil, always massaging from bottom to top, toward the heart. This is a time-consuming process and requires patience. Change the oils occasionally; instead of cypress, use lavender, rosemary, yarrow, or juniper, because they are also suited to application to the skin.

It's also advisable to take garlic capsules at the same time or to use a lot of fresh garlic in cooking. What's more, you should put your feet up, preferably higher than your head, about 10 minutes a day. Walking and swimming are beneficial, as well, because they encourage the function of the veins in the legs.

Demands are made on your skin every day, so it needs regular care. Pamper yourself daily with scented oils.

Skin Care

It has been said that we are only as old as we feel. This is true, in a sense, but we are also as old as we look—to other people anyway. But fortunately there is a lot we can do to combat the outward signs of aging.

❧ In a healthy, young body, cells regenerate after a short period of time—anywhere from a few days to a few months. In the body of an older person, however, cell regeneration takes longer. But there are essential oils that older people can use that will stimulate cell regeneration, such as lavender, neroli, and patchouli. Vetiver will encourage the regeneration of the hypodermic tissue.

❧ Burst veins will usually disappear from the cheeks after rubbing on a blend of 10 ml of jojoba oil and 1 drop of real rose oil.

❧ For cleansing the face, myrtle oil is suitable for most skin types (except for very dry skin); rosewater from your pharmacy or health food store should be used simultaneously.

∞ Lavender water works particularly well for dry and irritated skin. One drop of lavender oil in half a quart, or liter, of distilled water will be sufficient.

∞ Dry, rough skin is best cared for with almond oil, blended with a little benzoin, nerol, and orange. Ylang-ylang will provide further nourishment and moisture for the skin.

∞ You can blend your own wrinkle-reducing facial oils and creams by using the essential oils of carrot seed, myrrh, neroli, and frankincense. They will also prevent further wrinkles from appearing. The best carrier oils for this purpose are avocado and jojoba, but it's advisable to also add 25 percent wheat germ oil. For the cream, I recommend a completely plant-based and fragrance-free cream base. Carefully stir in a little wheat germ oil before you add the essential oils.

Rejuvenating All Skin Types

Take advantage of these remedies, if you want optimal care for aging skin that will keep it looking young for a long time. Don't be afraid to experiment a little to discover "your" bath and massage oils, and "your" additions to cosmetics. Coordinate your perfume with these oils. You will find further hints and advice in "Tips for the Correct Use Of Aroma Oils."

Looking good as you advance in years will also protect you from feeling resigned and bitter. It will boost your self-confidence, show that you are active and enjoying life, and release powers that you never knew you had. A fresh look is especially attractive in older people, and this doesn't take witchcraft, but just a little extra care with your skin.

To keep your skin looking young, use facial toners, creams, and oils, with neroli and rose, which are suitable for all skin types. Dilute these oils in a carrier oil that is high in fat to ensure good skin care. Both oils are also beneficial for chapped skin that is prone to inflammation.

REMEDY

A SPECIAL OIL FOR AGING SKIN

Blend 3 drops each of vetiver, patchouli, and bitter orange (or ylang-ylang) and 1 drop of neroli (very expensive, so alternatively use petit-grain) with 30 ml of almond oil in a bottle. Shake well and leave to mature in the refrigerator for 14 days. Use as a night cream.

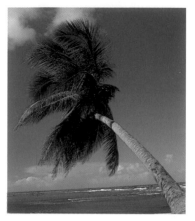

Going on vacation? Don't forget your essential oils!

Aromatherapy at Home and on Vacation

A few annoying mosquitoes in the bedroom, a line of ants meandering through the bungalow, blisters on tired feet, and a painful sunburn—all this can spoil the best weeks of the year for us. However, if you take the right essential oils with you on vacation, you will have nothing to worry about. At home, too, aromatherapy helps us cope with all sorts of irritating problems.

Relief for Allergies

Allergies, such as asthma, eczema, hay fever, and nettle rash, can occur for many reasons, at home and on vacation. Some are caused by chemicals in our food, whereas others are a reaction to pollen from certain grasses and trees. If you suffer from allergies, it's advisable to discuss them with your doctor before you go on a vacation.

Nettle Rash

Lukewarm baths with 3 drops each of chamomile and melissa have produced the best results for nettle rash. If only small areas of the skin are affected, cold compresses will be sufficient. Fill a large bowl with boiled cold water,

The fresh, lemon-like scent of melissa not only refreshes and revives, but also alleviates allergic reactions. Its antiviral properties are successfully utilized in treating allergies, such as hay fever. In addition, its strengthening effect improves the overall condition of people suffering from allergies.

and add 2 drops of lavender or melissa, stirring thoroughly. Repeated baths and compresses every few hours are recommended until the red wheals have disappeared.

Hay Fever

Rose oil, which is very expensive, has been proven to be very effective in treating hay fever. Fortunately, there are less costly alternatives: eucalyptus, chamomile, lavender, and melissa.

Soothing Blisters

If you have gotten blisters on your feet after a long walk, carefully dab on some undiluted lavender oil. Alternatively, use benzoin or peru balsam.

Help for an Upset Stomach

Unusual food abroad can easily give rise to Montezuma's Revenge, and not just in Latin America. Often the culprit is water that hasn't been boiled used in local restaurants for washing fruit and vegetables and making ice cream. Taking garlic capsules or plenty of fresh garlic is the best preventive measure.

Healing Frostbite

People on winter vacation, or anyone who stays out in the freezing cold too long, are susceptible to frostbite. To treat the itchiness and the pain, rub on a massage oil containing 3 percent each of marjoram and pepper oil. The essen-

IMPORTANT
Don't treat children with peppermint oil unless they are at least six years old.

If your bowels rebel:

❧ **Apply warm compresses with chamomile, lavender, myrrh, rosemary, thyme, and/or juniper to the abdomen.**

❧ **Drink plenty of warm peppermint tea. Once the acute symptoms have subsided, also drink mineral water fortified with lemon.**

TIP
Do not apply essential oils to frostbite that has already burst open.

Put together your own "essential" first-aid travel kit well in time for a business trip or a vacation.

tial oils of geranium, chamomile, rose, juniper, and lemon also have a good reputation for healing frostbite. The simplest and often most effective method is to inhale the scent straight from the bottle. Some people find steam inhalations beneficial, although others find that the heat exacerbates their complaints. You will have to experiment to see which method works best for you. Cold compresses with either rosewater or chamomile tea are a tonic for red, inflamed eyes.

Chasing Away Insects and Treating Insect Bites

Ants, Fleas, and Lice

TIP
Just as citrus oils keep annoying insects at bay, you can also use them to protect your furniture from being scratched by your cat. Simply polish the furniture with a little citronella oil.

Ants do not like lavender, sandalwood, or tea tree oil. If you place 2 or 3 drops in front of their hole, they will soon look for another playground. Wiping the threshold with a little lavender oil will keep them at bay as well. However, ants are very useful creatures, so you should just chase them away. Do not put essential oils in their nests.

Both humans and their pets can be freed of fleas with

Protecting Pets from Fleas

🌱 Spread 2 to 3 drops of lavender oil in your palms.

🌱 Don't forget your pet's sides and tummy.

🌱 Stroke your dog or cat from head to tail, thereby spreading the scent from your hands.

the help of lavender and lemon oil. For humans, baths and rubs are advisable. It's also helpful to scent clothing. Lice will run for cover if you rub your head thoroughly with one of the following oils: bergamot, eucalyptus, camphor, lavender, rosemary, or thyme. Rosemary oil is strongly recommended, because it is said to encourage hair growth, and thyme is said to work even better in this respect. A few drops are sufficient, although you will have to repeat the treatment.

Moths

Our great-grandmothers knew that moths can't bear the smell of lavender. This is why they hung little sachets filled with dried lavender flowers in their wardrobes. Add a few drops of lavender oil onto the sachets, which are back in fashion today, and this will increase the effect. When you are wiping out your wardrobes and drawers, add a few drops of lavender or cedar oil to a damp cloth. Moths also flee from the scents of cajeput, eucalyptus, myrtle, and tea tree. In addition to damaging clothing, moths can be found in food.

Mosquitoes, Wasps, and Bees

If you take a bottle of lavender or tea tree oil with you on trips or vacations, you won't have to worry about insect bites any longer. Regardless of whether you have been bitten by a mosquito or stung by a wasp or a bee, just apply a few drops to the bite immediately and repeat every few minutes until the itching has subsided. Sometimes the itching recurs after 24 hours, but this won't be a problem, because you will have the treatment with you. Basil, cajeput, melissa, and lemon will also provide instant relief, as long as you don't scratch.

Bergamot is a fruit produced from crossing lemon with bitter orange. Its oil has a pleasantly fruity scent and a reviving effect. Its antiseptic and disinfectant properties help alleviate head lice and prevent the scalp from producing excessive oil or dandruff.

It's helpful to use lavender oil right away if you get bit or stung by an insect. It dulls the pain, prevents inflammation, and has a relaxing effect on the entire body.

REMEDY

RUB FOR STIFF MUSCLES
(from R. Tisserand)

Blend 10 drops of rosemary, 6 drops of lemongrass, and 9 drops of juniper with 50 ml of vegetable oil. Rub onto the affected parts.

The fresh, reviving scent of peppermint provides quick help in alleviating dizziness, a racing heart, nervous excitement, and faintness. You can also use the oil for gentle massages to relieve headaches or a stiff neck.

Protection from Fleas and Mosquitoes

The following oils will keep these pests at a distance. Add at least 20 drops to the water in your essence burner.

Basil	Eucalyptus	Lemon
Cedar	Geranium	Lemongrass
Clove	Melissa	Peppermint

Soothing Sore Muscles

Stiff muscles can be loosened with chamomile, lavender, marjoram, and juniper. In hot countries, rubs with peppermint oil diluted in jojoba or another vegetable oil will have a cooling and very soothing effect.

Travel First Aid

❧ Excitement: If nervous excitement over an upcoming trip outweighs joyful anticipation, it is best dampened with benzoin, cananga, geranium, jasmine, chamomile, melissa, neroli, rose, sandalwood, or vetiver. Inhale the scent from the bottle every now and then, and also have it handy when the trip begins.

❧ Travel sickness: If you know from experience that you easily become travel sick, it's advisable to take some melissa, neroli, rose, or sandalwood with you; basil, lavender, and peppermint also work well. Lavender oil, best used in a spray, is well suited to improve the air quality in a train compartment, in the car, or on a plane. Another option is to take along little clay jugs of the oil.

These jugs are sealed with a cork, and the scent will remain for weeks, perhaps even months.

❧ Tiredness: Eucalyptus, grapefruit, lemongrass, lime, and lemon will refresh you if you are tired. All five will also improve the air quality instantly.

❧ Infection: You will be in contact with a lot of people on a train, boat, or plane trip. To reduce the possible risk of infection, it's advisable to carry an essential oil that will kill bacteria and viruses. Rosemary and tea tree oil are best, but basil and thyme also serve this purpose.

Cooling Sunburn

Lavender and peppermint oil diluted in jojoba or another vegetable oil help to soothe sunburn when dabbed onto the affected skin. If blisters have already formed, you can apply lavender undiluted. Lukewarm baths with 5 to 6 drops of chamomile oil or 6 drops of lavender oil added to 2 tablespoons of jojoba oil and 1 tablespoon of honey will also provide quick relief.

Eucalyptus, lemongrass, lime, mint, and lemon have disinfectant and refreshing effects, and are good to use in rooms where there are a lot of people. Jojoba oil is an ancient Native American remedy used to treat skin complaints and inflammations. It can also be used in hair care. Containing the most important vitamins, jojoba nourishes the skin and is suitable for all skin types. It also provides protection from sunlight (factor 4) and even helps to maintain a tan for longer.

REMEDY

SUNBURN LOTION

Blend 12 drops of lavender with 1 tablespoon of cooled boiled water. Shake well and dab onto the affected skin.

Your "Essential" First-Aid Travel Kit

❦ 1 bottle of lavender oil (to improve air quality and treat sunburn)

❦ 1 bottle of rosemary oil (to alleviate exhaustion and prevent infections)

❦ 1 bottle of peppermint oil (refreshes, fights headaches, and prevents mosquito bites)

❦ 1 bottle of tea tree oil (to treat infections, and for disinfecting)

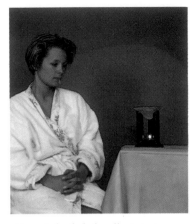

Essential oils help alleviate insomnia, inner restlessness, and nightmares.

Frankincense is good to use for calming the nerves, because its spicy, woody scent makes us feel peaceful and in harmony. It also has pain-reducing, anti-spasmodic, and anti-inflammatory properties, which are useful in treating colds.

How to Sleep Like a Baby

More and more people today complain of insomnia and restless sleep. There can be a variety of causes: a stressful job, family problems, worries and fears (see "Harmonizing Scents"), lack of exercise, or the common problem of being unable to switch off from the concerns of a busy day. Some people have trouble letting go of their thoughts, and become further and further entangled in them.

If sleeplessness persists for several weeks or more, you will enter a vicious circle. As you worry about not being able to fall asleep, it will become more and more difficult to do so.

Nervousness and Restlessness

If you experience nervousness and an inner restlessness without an obvious cause—in other words, if they are not related to stress—this usually means that there is a weakness in your nervous system. But you will be glad to know that essential oils can have a very positive influence on the nervous system, when used in baths, massage oils, and cosmetics, and for scenting rooms.

Bergamot, camphor, marjoram, melissa, orange, and chamomile have a soothing and balancing effect on the nerves. Angelica, basil, geranium, mandarin, petitgrain, and vetiver have a strengthening, restoring effect, and are especially helpful for people who are emotionally strained and weakened.

Insomnia and Nightmares

A relaxing aroma bath (not too hot) in the evening is a good and harmless sleeping aid. However, don't rush it, take your time, switch off, and enjoy. And don't take that horror novel to bed with you afterward.

Essential oils that promote relaxation are all suitable (see the list on page 78). Choose from these oils the ones that are right for you, and create your own blends. For a full bath, a total of 12 to 15 drops of oil are sufficient. Take extra care, however, when using melissa, thyme, and bergamot. Never add more than 3 drops of them.

Scenting your bedroom in the correct way also plays an important role. It's even more effective if you add the respective oils to your essence burner in the living room earlier in the evening. And don't eat sweets before bedtime, because the sugar will keep you awake. Drink a cup of chamomile tea instead.

Cedar, lavender, rose, jasmine, bergamot, and sandalwood, added to the essence burner, will aid restful sleep. Alternatively, a drop of cedar, lavender, and rose on your pillow will help you drift off faster.

TIP
If you use clary sage in your bath, avoid drinking alcohol before and after, because this could cause nightmares.

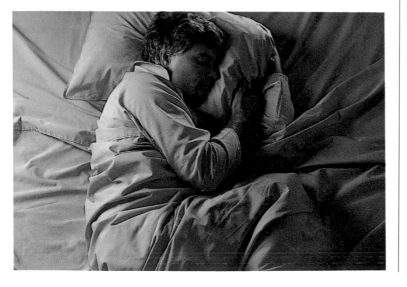

Falling asleep and sleeping through the night are increasing problems for many people today. Scenting your bedroom with the right essential oils will have a calming and relaxing effect, and will create a healthy atmosphere for you to sleep in.

REMEDY

A RELAXING BATH

Add 2 drops of neroli, 3 drops of bergamot, and 5 drops of lavender to approximately 150 ml of cream, and pour into a full bath.

The essential oil of clary sage creates feelings of euphoria and provides inspiration. Aromatherapy uses this oil to treat tension, fear, depression, and melancholy. Clary sage inspires creative people, as it gives rise to exceptional ideas.

Essential Oils for Relaxation

Benzoin	Juniper	Petitgrain
Bergamot	Lavender	Rose
Chamomile	Marjoram	Rosewood
Clary sage	Melissa	Sandalwood
Frankincense	Neroli	Spikenard
Geranium	Orange	Ylang-ylang

If you don't see the desired results immediately, do not despair; sometimes such changes take time to manifest. Try out different oils until you find the ones that help you the most. Trust your nose completely. I have seen good results with benzoin, lavender, orange, and sandalwood.

If you suffer from nightmares, your first choice should be melissa, neroli, and sandalwood. Alternatively, you might try petitgrain, rose, and frankincense, especially for scenting the bedroom.

If You Are Overwrought and Feeling Stressed

Being overwrought is usually caused by excessive demands being made on your body and mind. A common response to such a situation is anger, and anger and stress can often lead to troubled sleep. If you try to compensate with social drugs, such as alcohol, caffeine, or nicotine, you will only exacerbate the problem.

Angelica, geranium, clary sage, rosemary, and thyme all strengthen the body's defenses in stressful situations, but they do not necessarily aid sleep. Taking a warm bath in the evening, with honey oil, chamomile, lavender, marjoram, melissa, neroli, rose, or ylang-ylang, will be more beneficial.

Sorrow and Grief

It's very difficult to escape your sorrows and sad thoughts when you are lying in your bed feeling exhausted. Often it is at that time that pain really hits. For example, you may be thinking about the passing on of a friend or about a relationship that has come to an end, and this is keeping you from being able to drift off into a refreshing, restful sleep. Another vicious circle begins: The more exhausted we are, the more susceptible we are to being overwhelmed by the sorrow and grief in our lives. As a remedy for such a situation, before you go to bed, spray your bedroom with a mixture of water, some pure alcohol, and about 5 percent of the respective essential oils (see the list of mood-lifting oils below). Jasmine and ylang-ylang should not, however, dominate the blend.

You can also add these oils to a diffuser or aroma stone on your bedside table. Or, you can inhale the scent of your favorite oil directly from the bottle. Try to let the lovely scent comfort you and help you switch off. It may be helpful to remember that nothing in life is permanent and that better times lie ahead.

We all have to learn to cope with grief, because life doesn't consist of sunny days only. But try to look ahead with optimism.

Mood-Lifting Essential Oils

Benzoin	Geranium	Orange
Bergamot	Grapefruit	Peru balsam
Camphor	Jasmine	Rose
Cedar	Lavender	Rosewood
Chamomile	Melissa	Sandalwood
Clary sage	Neroli	Ylang-ylang

How to Release Your Mental Powers

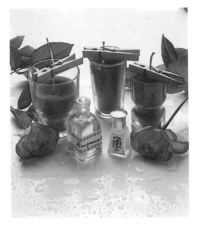

Scented candles stimulate the mind and the body

By being creative, you will express what is yours entirely, your special individuality. Accept that you are unique!

There is scarcely an essential oil that will not stimulate the mind in some way. It has been said that Napoleon literally poured rosemary water over himself every morning, to refresh and prepare himself for a stressful day ahead. If you wish to imitate Napoleon, add 2 drops of rosemary to cold water, or prepare a face and body formula with 5 drops of rosemary and 2 drops of stone pine in 100 ml of distilled water. Supposedly the German poet Schiller was inspired by the aroma of apples rotting in his desk drawer. Perhaps the smell reminded him of some long-forgotten childhood experience.

I walked past a sawmill every day on my way to school when I was a child, and even today I feel revived by the scent of freshly sawn wood.

Creativity

Creativity is not a privilege limited to artists. Anyone can be creative, and in many different ways and areas. Take, for example, arranging flowers, making children's toys, and playing the guitar; these are all creative activities. Let the scents of your choice put you in the right mood to unleash your creativity.

Feel free to try out scents other than those traditionally believed to promote creativity. Everyone reacts to scents in a different way. Add a few drops of your favorite oil to the essence burner or the room spray, use this oil to scent your cosmetics, or blend the "Creative" perfume (for the formula, turn to "Tips for the Correct Use of Aroma Oils").

Essential Oils That Promote Creativity

Cinnamon	Hyssop	Rose
Clary sage	Iris	Verbena

Inspiration

Not only do intellectual endeavors require inspiration, but you also have to be able to concentrate on the task at hand. Peppermint, rosemary, and thyme promote mental clarity and the ability to concentrate. If you are overflowing with ideas but have trouble organizing them, angelica will help you curb the onrush. Cedar and cypress will also lead you back into the world of what is possible and attainable.

A blend of several inspiring essential oils is particularly effective. Why don't you try a few drops of bergamot, rosemary, sandalwood, and lemon or lemongrass oil in your

To have new ideas is one side of the coin, and to be able to structure them and apply them realistically is the other. The key is obtaining the right balance, just like when you are blending scents.

Essential Oils That Encourage Inspiration

Bergamot	Lemon	Rosemary
Clary sage	Lemongrass	Savory
Coriander	Petitgrain	Sandalwood

You may be surprised at how much essential oils can strengthen your self-confidence and your faith in your own success.

essence burner? Clary sage harmonizes well with bergamot and cypress, which also aid concentration. Using peppermint oil can be a little tricky, because the scent is quite dominant, but it goes well with verbena, rosemary, and lemon.

Self-confidence

When you want to work creatively, it helps to have a healthy sense of your own worth. If you don't believe in yourself, it will be difficult to achieve anything. The respective essential oils (see the list below) will help you mobilize your hidden powers and give you greater self-confidence.

The fresh, dry scent of bay oil has a stimulating and mood-lifting effect on the entire system. Because of its antiseptic properties, bay oil is added to a number of medicines.

In the beginning, however, what is most important is not to set your aims too high. Not everybody wielding a brush will become another Rembrandt. But that is not the point anyway. It's important for creative work to have a playful element—in other words, it should be fun. It should also entail the desire to try something new, and to explore one's possibilities, while also becoming aware of one's limitations.

Essential Oils That Boost Self-confidence

Angelica	Grapefruit	Petitgrain
Basil	Juniper	Rosemary
Bay	Neroli	Sage
Bergamot	Nutmeg	Thuja
Cypress	Patchouli	Thyme

One aspect of creative work is knowing when it is time to give it a rest or finish it. If you tend to become overzealous, then bay, clary sage, neroli, and petitgrain will help you let go, or find your way out of the maze you have constructed for yourself. These oils will also help you find new joy in your creativity, and give you new stimuli. On the other hand, if you find it difficult to begin a creative project, the scents of angelica, bay, nutmeg, rosemary, and sage will give you the confidence that is needed to take the first step.

Meditation

For thousands of years, people in religious communities have used scents to achieve inner calm and to establish better contact with the spiritual world. Among the "holy" scents are elemi, myrrh, peru balsam, rose, sandalwood, juniper, frankincense, hyssop, and cedar. Adding just 1 or 2 drops of all these oils to your essence burner will result in an exciting fusion of scents. Of course, you may want to use only a few of these oils, but it shouldn't be less than three, if possible. However, there are others as well:

❧ Benzoin is particularly suited to people who are under a lot of emotional stress.

❧ Styrax has a balancing effect on people who are irritable and have shown a tendency to become hysterical.

❧ Thuja allows a stressed person to take a healing break, to rethink a situation, and it also fosters new strength.

❧ Cypress helps us concentrate on the essential.

These "holy" scents cleanse the body and the soul, and expand the mind. They open a channel in the soul for God's order and harmony. If you like to meditate alone or with friends, you will find that when these oils are used in an essence burner they provide a gentle support.

The simplest form of meditation consists of consciously focusing the mind on the flow of breath in and out of the body. Essential oils, such as benzoin, styrax, thuja, and cypress, can help to make a meditative state more accessible.

The oldest perfume on record is "Kyphi," an incense blend from Egypt. Its ingredients are recorded on the Papyrus Eberus (1550 B.C.). It contains 16 different components, including frankincense and myrrh. Writers of the period mention its antispasmodic and calming effects and its ability to alleviate fear and panic.

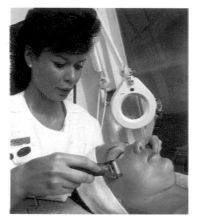

Essential oils are well suited for use in cosmetics.

Tips for the Correct Use of Aroma Oils

Now comes the magic. Here, you will learn how to blend your own scents, which will be unmistakably yours. There is no limit to the possibilities. Every blend of aroma oils will result in an entirely new scent. But it's important to pay attention to dosages. Adding one drop more or less can produce a different scent. Try it!

All scents fit into one of the following three categories: top note, middle note, and base note. Top note describes a fresh, light, and clear scent, which develops quickly, but evaporates just as fast. Middle note refers to a full-bodied, sweet scent, which appeals to our emotions. Base note refers to earthy, warm scents, which are obtained from woods and roots, and are long lasting.

Always keep to the recommended dosage. Less can be more in aromatherapy.

Basic Rules

Essence burner: Fill the bowl with water, and add 5 to 8 drops of the essential oil, and then stir. Light the candle underneath the bowl. Replenish the water from time to time. The bowl can be cleaned with hot water and vinegar.

Diffuser and aroma stone: Simply drip the essential oil on—just a few drops are enough. Clean with hot water only and let dry.

You can use essential oils in various ways. Which way is best depends on many different factors. Bear your own personal experience in mind.

Scent jug: Add a few drops of the essential oil, and then close firmly.

Mist spray: A mist-spray bottle made of glass, porcelain, or ceramic works best. Fill with distilled water or noncarbonated mineral water, pure alcohol, and 3 to 5 drops of the essential oil. Close and shake.

Steam inhalation: Fill a large bowl with hot water, and add a few drops of the aroma oil. Bend over the bowl, draping a bath towel over your head and shoulders so that the steam can't escape. Breathe in calmly for 5 to 10 minutes.

Baths: For a full bath, 15 to 20 drops of the essential oil will be sufficient. Stir them into 1 to 2 tablespoons of cream, whey, full milk, runny honey, or liquid soap. You can also use the same amount of vegetable oil (peanut, thistle, almond, avocado or jojoba). The addition of an emulsifier (such as liquid lecithin) will render the oil blend hydrophilic, which basically means that it will dissolve in water. Turn on the faucets, and pour the blend into the water, and then stir. For hip baths, use 10 to 12 drops of the essential oil; for foot baths, 5 to 8 drops.

It's important to remember the strength of the different oils. Hot water, for example, increases the effects of citrus oils and of rosemary oil, so care should be taken when using these oils in baths.

Body and facial oils (also for massages and rubs): Use 50 ml of jojoba or almond oil as a carrier oil. For aging or very dry skin, add 10 percent of wheat germ oil; for impure skin, add 2 to 3 drops of tea tree oil. Next add 15 to 20 drops of your chosen essential oils, and shake well. For children, 5 to 7 drops will be sufficient; for babies, 1 drop is enough.

TIP
Never use aggressive soaps when taking an aroma bath. Essential oils do not react well with them.

Because of the soothing warmth of the water and the healing powers of the essential oils, a bath affects all aspects of our being. For a morning bath, choose stimulating oils (rosemary, thyme, verbena); in the evening, use relaxing, harmonizing oils (ylang-ylang, chamomile, lavender).

Observe carefully how your skin reacts to a blend. This will help you find the remedy that is ideally suited to you.

Jojoba oil is obtained from the seeds of the jojoba bush, which is native to Central America. It works well as a base for cosmetics, because it doesn't turn rancid.

Healing oils: The best carrier oils are aloe vera for sunburns and skin complaints; calendula for babies and toddlers and for sore muscles; St John's wort for inflammations, lumbago, rheumatism, and burns; jojoba for allergies, skin problems, menstrual complaints, and cellulite; and almond for circulatory problems and sore muscles. Dosages as for body oils, above.

Skin cream: Carefully stir 15 to 20 drops of the essential oils into 50 ml of a cream base.

Facial toner: Drip 2 to 3 drops of the essential oil (one type only) into 1 quart, or liter, of distilled water or non-carbonated mineral water. You can also add 1 tablespoon of pure alcohol. Shake well.

Perfume: You can choose between an oil- or an alcohol-based perfume. For an oil-based perfume, use 15 to 20 drops of the essential oils in about 10 ml of jojoba oil. For an alcohol-based perfume, mix 10 ml of pure alcohol (90

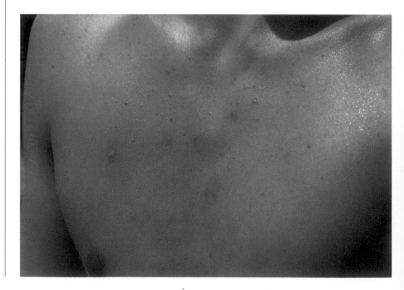

percent) with 50 to 100 percent of distilled water; then add 10 to 15 drops of the essential oils. Perfumes should be left to mature for a few weeks before being used. If you favor the most expensive scents (hyacinth, jasmine, neroli, and rose), fill the bottle in which the oil came with alcohol and water, or with jojoba oil. With thicker, more resinous oils, such as benzoin, use alcohol only.

Shampoo: Add 15 to 20 drops of the essential oil to 100 ml of a shampoo base.

The skin, in particular, deserves to be pampered with essential oils.

The Right Scents for Different Skin and Hair Types

Normal skin: Chamomile, geranium, jasmine, lavender, lemon, neroli, orange, rose, ylang-ylang (1 drop only).

Oily skin: Bergamot, camphor, lavender, lemongrass, petitgrain, rosemary, thyme, verbena, ylang-ylang.

Dry skin: Benzoin, cananga, chamomile, honey oil, lavender, neroli, palmarosa, rosewood, vetiver, ylang-ylang.

Sensitive skin: Chamomile, hyssop lavender, melissa, rosemary, sandalwood, yarrow.

Oily hair: Cedar, cypress lavender, lemon, melissa, sage.

Dry hair: Geranium, honey oil, rosemary, rosewood, ylang-ylang.

Dandruff: Cypress, eucalyptus, juniper, tea tree.

To encourage hair growth: Rosemary, sage, thyme.

Special shampoos with aroma oils can make your hair stronger and are good for the scalp. There are also formulas to treat specific problems, such as dandruff and head lice.

The Right Mix—Which Scents Work Together

You can also use your essential oil perfume to scent your cosmetics and bath oils.

❧ Lavender harmonizes with all other essential oils, with the exception of rosemary.

❧ All citrus oils can be blended without a problem, and they also go well with the oils obtained from coniferous trees.

❧ The characteristic scents of eucalyptus and peppermint can be enhanced with a few drops of lavender or rosemary.

❧ Flower oils usually harmonize with one another very well, too—take, for example, iris, jasmine, chamomile, lavender, neroli, rose, and ylang-ylang.

❧ Sandalwood, vetiver, cedar, or stone pine will create a more masculine note.

Aroma Oils for the Bath

Since ancient times, baths with essential oils were regarded as a luxury fit for kings and queens. In the Orient, in particular, people liked to indulge their senses in precious scents.

Bath oils can be used for different purposes and in a great variety of blends. There are a multitude of possible combinations; however, it's important to consult your doctor if you suffer from a specific complaint. What follow are a few suggestions for bath-oil blends.

Relaxation: Use 10 drops of sandalwood, 5 drops of bergamot, and 5 drops of lavender; 10 drops of lavender, 5 drops of neroli, and 5 drops of melissa; or 5 drops of chamomile, 5 drops of lavender, and 3 drops of vetiver. Geranium, honey oil, marjoram, rosewood, orange, and tonka bean will also provide restful sleep.

Stimulation: Use 5 drops of rosemary, 5 drops of petit-grain, 2 drops of peppermint, and 1 drop of lemon; 3 drops of thyme, 5 drops of verbena, 5 drops of myrtle, and 5 drops of lime; or 5 drops of angelica, 5 drops of juniper, 5 drops of petitgrain, and 3 drops of stone pine.

Skin care: Use 10 drops of sandalwood, 4 drops of chamomile, 4 drops of lavender, 1 drop of rose, and 1 drop of cedar; 5 drops of geranium, 2 drops of myrtle, 5 drops of orange, 5 drops of sandalwood, and 3 drops of frankincense; or 5 drops of benzoin, 3 drops of neroli, 3 drops of yarrow, 5 drops of sandalwood, and 3 drops of vetiver.

Creating an erotic mood: Use 5 drops of patchouli, 5 drops of sandalwood, 3 drops of vetiver, and 5 drops of ylang-ylang; or 5 drops of geranium, 5 drops of honey oil, 2 drops of jasmine, and 5 drops of peru balsam.

Scents have even been used by some department stores to influence the subconscious—it is hoped to an honorable end!

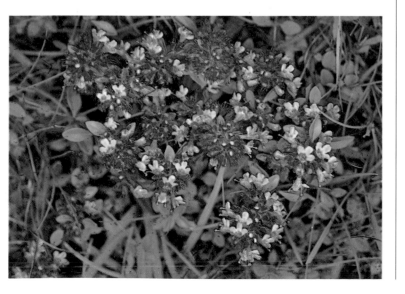

"Pick-me-up" thyme is one of the oils that has stimulating and anti-spasmodic effects. Thyme baths are recommended for the treatment of nervousness, rheumatic pain, swelling, and rickets.

Essential Oils for the Face and the Body

If you are making your own natural body and massage oils, you will need a carrier oil. This can come straight from your kitchen cupboard, as olive oil, sunflower oil, and wheat germ oil are particularly suitable.

For facial and skin creams, use 50 ml of a cream base, and stir in thoroughly the indicated amounts of essential oil blends. The following blends are also suitable for body massages and rubs.

Relaxation: Use jojoba oil with 3 drops of bergamot, 3 drops of lavender, 8 drops of sandalwood, and 5 drops of chamomile; or 5 drops of geranium, 3 drops of petitgrain, 5 drops of rosewood, 2 drops of rose, and 3 drops of cedar. Honey oil, coriander, mandarin, melissa, neroli, and orange also have a relaxing effect.

Sensual pleasure and healing can be close neighbors. Nature holds some mystifying and wonderful gifts for us.

For normal skin: Use 5 drops of geranium, 5 drops of lavender, 2 drops of neroli, 3 drops of orange, and 1 drop of ylang-ylang; or 2 drops of jasmine, 5 drops of

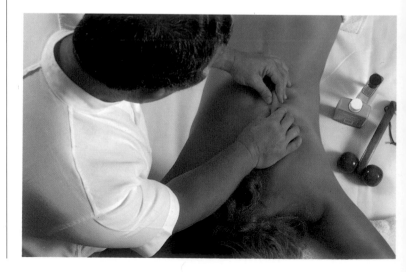

A massage oil that contains ginger, camphor, peppermint, and pepper oil will make a treatment twice as effective.

chamomile, 3 drops of lavender, 1 drop of rose, and 3 drops of sandalwood.

For oily skin: Use 5 drops of bergamot, 3 drops of verbena, 3 drops of petitgrain, 2 drops of thyme, and 2 drops of ylang-ylang; or 5 drops of lavender, 5 drops of lemongrass, 3 drops of rosemary, 2 drops of thyme, and 2 drops of myrtle.

For dry skin: Use 3 drops of benzoin, 3 drops of cananga, 5 drops of palmarosa, 3 drops of rosewood, and 3 drops of vetiver; or 5 drops of honey oil, 5 drops of chamomile, 3 drops of lavender, 2 drops of neroli, and 2 drops of ylang-ylang.

For sensitive skin: Use 5 drops of chamomile, 5 drops of melissa, 3 drops of rosemary, and 5 drops of yarrow; or 5 drops of chamomile, 5 drops of lavender, 5 drops of sandalwood, and 2 drops of hyssop.

For aging skin (and also to counteract wrinkles): Use 3 drops of benzoin, 5 drops of sandalwood, 3 drops of vetiver, 5 drops of frankincense, and 3 drops of ylang-ylang; or 5 drops of carrot seed, 3 drops of myrrh, 3 drops of neroli, and 5 drops of frankincense.

Essential Oil Facial Toners

Refreshing: Add 2 to 3 drops of myrtle or rosemary to 1 quart, or liter, of distilled water. You can also add some pure alcohol.

Relaxing: Add 2 to 3 drops of lavender or 1 drop of rose or neroli to the water and the alcohol.

Almond oil has been used for cosmetic purposes since ancient times. It maintains young and supple skin, and is suitable, just as jojoba oil is, for all skin types.

In creating your own perfume, always use small amounts to discover which scents produce a harmonious blend. Not only will your perfume give you your individual scent, but it will also influence your physical and mental well-being.

For every time of day: Add 2 to 3 drops of orange to the water and the alcohol.

Creating Your Own Perfume

Each perfume contains at least three different aroma oils: a warm base note, a light top note, and the middle note, which links the two others.

Oils suitable as base notes: Ambrette seed, benzoin, cinnamon, cedar, clove, cypress, elemi, frankincense, galbanum, honey oil, juniper, patchouli, pine, rosewood, sandalwood, stone pine, styrax, tonka bean, vetiver.

Oils suitable as top notes: Bergamot, lemon, lemongrass, lime, mandarin, orange, peppermint, verbena.

Oils suitable as middle notes: Chamomile, clary sage, geranium, hyssop, iris, jasmine, lavender, melissa, mimosa, myrtle, neroli, rose, tuberose, ylang-ylang.

A Few Fragrances to Get You Started

Perfume "Sylvia" (light and fresh): Blend 5 drops of frankincense, 1 drop of stone pine, 5 drops of myrtle, 3 drops of lime, 3 drops of orange, and 1 drop of peppermint oil.

Perfume "Sonya" (for the sporty type): Blend 5 drops of sandalwood, 2 drops of cypress, 3 drops of clary sage, 3 drops of myrtle, 3 drops of bergamot, 1 drop of pep-

Vetiver oil is obtained from the roots of the grass of the same name. It has a relaxing effect, especially on the nerves and on the female reproductive organs. It increases the likelihood of conceiving, and has a regulating effect on menstrual problems. Vetiver oil has an earthy, sweet scent and a viscous consistency, which is why it is used as a fixative for perfumes.

How to Create Your Personal Essential Oil Perfume

For your personal blend, use 10 to 30 drops of different essential oils (representing base, middle, and top notes) on 10 ml of jojoba oil.

1

First drip some of the base-note oil into the carrier oil (jojoba), checking the result on your skin.

2

Next add the middle-note oil, checking again. Add the top-note oil last.

3

Shake the mixture well after each addition.

4

If a certain scent prevails in the end, this can be balanced by adding a little more of one of the other oils that have been used in the blend. You could also add some lavender.

permint, and 1 drop of lemon.

Perfume "Giselle" (heavy and warm): Blend 5 drops of benzoin (dissolved in some pure alcohol), 10 drops of sandalwood, 3 drops of frankincense, 2 drops of ylang-ylang, and 3 drops of orange.

"Creative" perfume: Blend 10 drops of sandalwood, 2 drops of yarrow, 2 drops of cinnamon, 3 drops of iris, 1 drop of rose, and 5 drops of lemongrass.

Perfume "Julia" (erotic): Blend 3 drops of patchouli, 8 drops of sandalwood, 3 drops of jasmine, 1 drop of rose, 3 drops of ylang-ylang, and 3 drops of verbena.

If perfumes are stored in a cool, dark place, they will keep for a very long time. Many scents even improve with time if they are stored well.

Perfume for fearful people: Blend 3 drops of benzoin, 8 drops of sandalwood, 2 drops of patchouli, 5 drops of chamomile, 5 drops of ylang-ylang, and 5 drops of bergamot.

Perfume for anorexic people: Blend 8 drops of honey oil, 3 drops of jasmine or lavender, 1 drop of rose, 3 drops of ylang-ylang, 5 drops of bergamot, 3 drops of mandarin, and 3 drops of grapefruit.

Perfume for men: Blend 3 drops of sandalwood, 2 drops of juniper or 1 drop of styrax, 1 drop of vetiver, 3 drops of myrtle, 2 drops of lavender, 4 drops of bergamot, and 1 drop of lemon.

Before using any of these perfumes, store them in a cupboard for two to four weeks.

All perfumes need to mature in order to attain their full aroma . Allow about four weeks for your creation to develop a rounded, harmonious scent.

About This Book

About the Author

Gisela Bulla lives and works as a writer in Munich, Germany. She has published several books on a variety of subjects, and has studied aromatherapy intensively for many years.

Photo Credits

Elke Stolt Bildagentur, Ahrensburg: 1 (Michael Luft), 30 (Visualis), 76 (Matthias Stotlt), 90 (N.N.); Fotoarchiv, Essen: 54 (N.N.), 70 (Toma Babovic), 84 (Swapan Parekh), 86 (Bernd Euler); IFA-Bilderteam, Taufkirchen: 6 (Ventura), 13 (Borodulin), 35 (Göss-Holz), 51(Forkel), 62 (J. Heron), 77 (Comnet), 89 (Lederer); Kerth, Ulrich: cover, 17, 80; Mauritius, Mittenwald: 48 (Hubatka), N.N.: 94; Neumond-Düfte der Natur, Herrsching: 61; Rehm, Claudia, Stockdorf: 20; Tony Stone, München: 8 (Wilfried Krecichworst), 40 (Ian Shaw), 67 (Christopher Bissell); Zuche, Michael, München:19

Our thanks to the Neumond-Düfte der Natur GmbH in Herrsching, Germany, for helping to make this book possible.

Index